D1603085

ESSENTIAL OILS
&
AROMATHERAPY

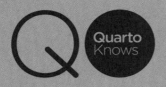

Inspiring | Educating | Creating | Entertaining

Brimming with creative inspiration, how-to projects, and useful
information to enrich your everyday life, Quarto Knows is a favorite
destination for those pursuing their interests and passions. Visit our
site and dig deeper with our books into your area of interest:
Quarto Creates, Quarto Cooks, Quarto Homes, Quarto Lives,
Quarto Drives, Quarto Explores, Quarto Gifts, or Quarto Kids.

First published in 2018 by Wellfleet Press,
an imprint of The Quarto Group
142 West 36th Street, 4th Floor
New York, NY 10018 USA
T (212) 779-4972 **F** (212) 779-6058
www.QuartoKnows.com

Wellfleet Press titles are also available at discount for retail, wholesale, promotional, and bulk purchase.
For details, contact the Special Sales Manager by email at specialsales@quarto.com or by mail at
The Quarto Group, Attn: Special Sales Manager, 401 Second Avenue North, Suite 310,
Minneapolis, MN 55401, USA.

10 9 8 7 6 5 4 3 2

ISBN: 978-1-57715-178-4

Cover and Interior Design: Ashley Prine, Tandem Books

Printed in China

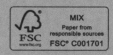

This book provides general information on various widely known and widely accepted images that tend
to evoke feelings of strength and confidence. However, it should not be relied upon as recommending or
promoting any specific diagnosis or method of treatment for a particular condition, and it is not intended
as a substitute for medical advice or for direct diagnosis and treatment of a medical condition by a
qualified physician. Readers who have questions about a particular condition, possible treatments for that
condition, or possible reactions from the condition or its treatment should consult a physician or other
qualified healthcare professional.

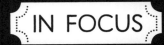

IN FOCUS

ESSENTIAL OILS & AROMATHERAPY

Your Personal Guide

MARLENE HOUGHTON, PhD

WELLFLEET
PRESS

CONTENTS

INTRODUCTION

"Their fruit will be for food and their
leaves for healing."

Ezekiel 47:12

Welcome to the fragrant art of aromatherapy. I have been using essential oils for many years for both health and beauty and have found them useful for the prevention and treatment of minor ailments and skin care. The life-enhancing qualities of this holistic system of medicine have provided my family and me with vital protection from colds, coughs, and flu during the winter months, and pleasure when used for skin and body care.

This ancient healing system has become very popular with the general public, and today many women's magazines carry articles on essential oils and their uses. Aromatherapy has left the fringes and become complementary to mainstream medicine. The aim of this book is to introduce the layperson to the principles of this wonderful therapy so that readers, armed with a broad knowledge of the basics of these essential oils and their application, will be able to gain many health benefits by using the oils for prevention, healing, beauty, and pleasure.

Many aromatherapy books concentrate on women and their health and beauty issues, but I thought it was time that men were also included. I have added a chapter on aromatherapy oils for men, as male skin is not the same as female skin, and men also have to deal with the daily ritual of shaving, which can be associated with a number of skin problems. This information seems to be hard for men to find, and they have been neglected, so I have attempted to put this right. At last there are some valuable tips for men when using aromatherapy that will help them with natural daily grooming. Male readers will recognize the benefits that these aromatic essences will bring to their skin, body, hair, and health when they start to use them, and they will wonder how they ever managed without them.

Aromatherapy Today

This form of ageless medicine used for thousands of years throughout Europe and the Far East has gained popularity in the West. Today it has become one of the most popular and fastest-growing branches of complementary medicine. Researchers and many medical professionals increasingly recognize aromatherapy's therapeutic value in helping to keep the body, mind, and spirit in harmony. Recognizing the healing properties of essential plant oils, practitioners trained today learn that this healing modality is a gentle holistic therapy that draws its powers from Mother Nature's plants, flowers, leaves, roots, seeds, fruits, and barks. Used to relieve stress, boost physical and psychological well-being, and improve the health of the immune system, this popular therapy is being used more and more by enlightened practitioners of mainstream medicine although it has not yet been accepted scientifically. The claims made for aromatherapy's healing effect according to science are not supported by any research or evidence. It is true that most of the evidence in favor of the use of essential oils for healing and prevention is empirical, gathered first-hand over centuries and through observation. The upsurge in interest in this holistic therapy, however, is due to the acceptance by the public of aromatherapy principles and skepticism regarding using only drugs to restore health.

I accept the wisdom of the ancients, and my experience when using these precious essential oils therapeutically has proven to me that they have preventative and restorative value. I think that over 8,000 years of use shows that Mother Nature's essential oils have withstood the test of time and that these plant oils play a valuable part in the treatment of minor ailments and also health problems that orthodox medicine is unable to cure.

Enclosed Essential Oil Wall Chart

Included in this book is a wall chart that serves as a quick and handy go-to reference guide containing a summary of the major essential oils, their characteristics, and their healing properties from the following pages.

Take Care Never drink any essential oil, whether diluted or not. Oils should be diluted in a carrier or base oil and massaged into the skin, put into bath water, or warmed in a diffuser to fill a room with a specific aroma. Some oils will require a patch test, which involves putting a little of the mixture on one spot on your arm to see if it causes an irritation.

❋ ❋ ❋

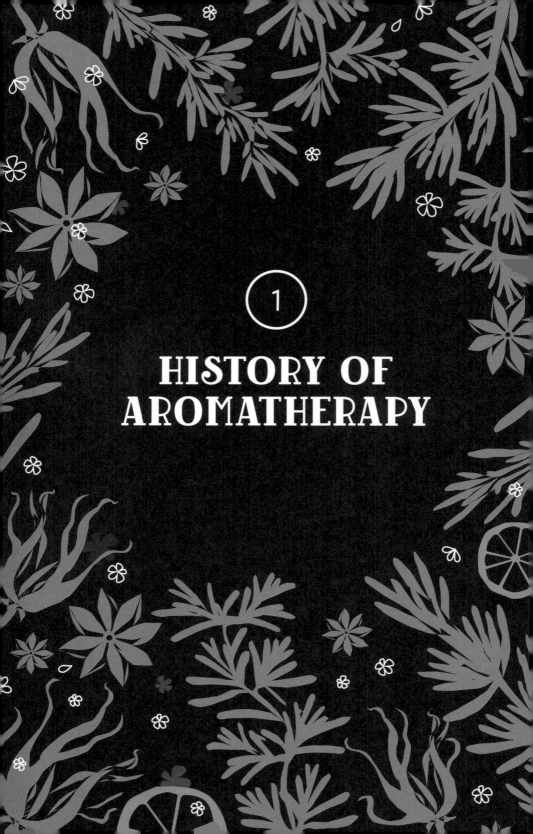

1

HISTORY OF AROMATHERAPY

*"But Flowers distilled though they with Winter meet,
lose but their show, their substance still lives sweet."*

William Shakespeare

Aromatherapy is the art of using essential oils for the purpose of restoring balance to the mind, body, and spirit. It is a form of natural healing that goes back more than 8,000 years. Many think that aromatherapy is a New Age therapy, but in fact it is one of the oldest known medicinal therapies. Like all other holistic treatments, it works on the principle that the most effective way to promote health and well-being is to strengthen the immune system, which is critically important to good health. This healing art is also good for stress reduction, as it promotes calm and balance, restoring the body and mind to a state of equilibrium. Aromatherapy treats the whole person: the physical body, the emotions, and the spirit. In this way, harmony is reinstated between this important team that makes up the whole person by bringing each system into alignment.

The application of essential oils for therapeutic purposes can be traced back to all major civilizations. In the ancient world perfumed oils, believed to be sacred, were used in rituals and religious ceremonies. They were also used medicinally by priests/physicians to treat many of the diseases that have afflicted humankind since the beginning of time.

In India this tradition has not been lost, and temples built entirely from sandalwood are still in existence. Ayurveda, the holistic tradition of medicine in India—over 3,000 years old—is practiced by present-day Ayurvedic doctors who still use traditional health care concepts when treating patients. Oil massage treatments for health and well-being are an important holistic therapy in Ayurvedic medicine. For relaxation of the body and mind, skin nourishment, improvement of circulation, and removal of toxins, Ayurveda uses many essential oils to good effect.

Ancient Chinese herbals going back thousands of years describe the use of aromatic woods and herbs that were burnt as offerings to the Gods. The essential oils from plants, barks, roots, leaves, and seeds were also used medicinally by Chinese apothecaries. In 2650 BCE, *The Yellow Emperor's Classic of Internal Medicine* contained references to these valuable oils.

The ancient Egyptians, regarded as the founders of this healing art, used therapeutic oils in massage, skin care, and medicinally. The High Priests burned heady mixtures made up of spikenard, cinnamon, and other rich and potent ingredients so that the Sun God Ra would return safely in the eastern skies every morning. They also used cedarwood and other aromatic oils for embalming the dead. Cedarwood was the wood of choice for the sarcophagi in which the royal Egyptian mummies were buried. In the Ebers Papyrus, dated 1550 BCE, medicinal formulas were found for various diseases that were treated with inhalations, compresses, and gargles. Essential oils are truly ancient medicine.

In the Middle East, merchants brought back precious spices, cinnamon, ginger, frankincense, and myrrh from their journeys to the Orient. Between the seventh and thirteenth centuries, the Arabs produced many scholars and scientists. An Arabian physician and philosopher born in Persia in 980 CE named Ibn Sina, and known more often as Avicenna, the Prince of Physicians, has been credited with the discovery of distillation, the method most commonly used to obtain the oils. This gifted man of science wrote more than a hundred books, and his book *The Canon of Medicine* was used by students of medicine

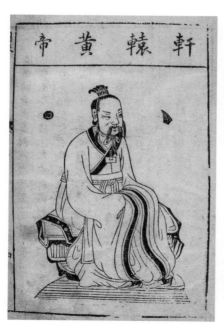

The Yellow Emperor

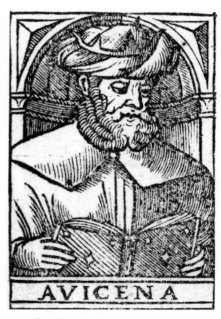

Ibn Sina, also known as Avicenna

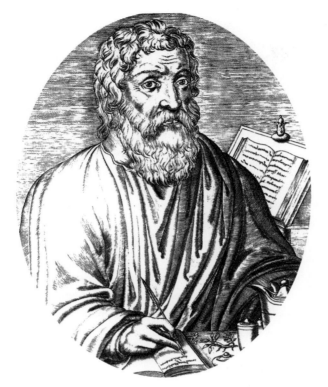

Hippocrates

for many centuries. One of his books was devoted entirely to the rose, the most valued flower of Islam, whose reavenly and divine fragrance is believed to have permeated the Garden of Allah. Legend has it that the ruby-red damask rose petals were created from a single drop of sweat from the brow of the Prophet.

The classical Greeks used these precious oils in their bath houses for relaxation, hygiene, health, and beauty. Hippocrates, the Greek physician who today is known as the Father of Medicine, advocated the benefits of bathing in warm baths scented with sweet-smelling perfumed oils. Later, the Romans obtained much of their medical knowledge of essential oils from the Greeks and then improved on this knowledge. They were aware of the beneficial properties of these wonderful oils and, apart from using them to treat disease, the Romans—well known for their hedonistic lifestyles—used them for sensual reasons, to enhance sexual desire and uplift and alter mood. Unfortunately, with the fall of the Roman Empire around 410 CE, the use of these valuable oils declined in Europe, probably as the influence of the Church began to get a grip. The Church frowned on pleasure-seeking practices, communal bathing, and using fragrance for beautifying the body, judging them to be sinful and vain. Consequently, the use of these beautiful essential oils, for pleasure and also for use medicinally, fell into decline. The lack of hygiene during the Dark Ages led to the rise of many diseases, and ultimately the plagues in which millions of people died.

During this time, when the bubonic plagues wreaked havoc throughout Europe, herbalist-physicians urged people to use essential oils in an effort to stop the outbreaks from spreading. When they treated their patients, they wore beaked masks filled with cloves, cinnamon, and aromatic spices, believing that breathing the herbal aroma through this beak would protect them. They must have looked terrifying in this hideous outfit, and many of the victims probably died of fright instead of bubonic plague!

These plague-doctors carried sponges soaked in aromatic oils for protection but unfortunately this did not appear to work and thousands died. However, one group of people was protected against these epidemics, and it was not known why. They used what came to be known as "Four Thieves Vinegar." It contained many herbs and oils and appeared to provide protection against the infection. The name derived from a story about four thieves who robbed the dead victims of the plague. They doused themselves in this vinegar and mysteriously did not appear to catch this virulent disease that was killing millions. One of the therapeutic ingredients in this vinegar was garlic. Today we know that this pungent, volatile garlic oil contains important antibacterial and antiviral properties. 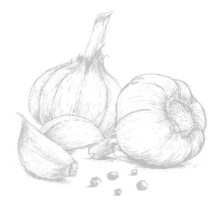 Other essential oils in this protective mixture were rosemary, eucalyptus, and cinnamon. These oils contain substances that obviously helped defend the four thieves from catching the pestilence. Today we know that these three essential oils are strongly antiseptic, and this must have been the reason these thieves did not die. Who said crime does not pay!

In Tudor England, Elizabeth I (1533–1603) used fragrant oils to cover what must have been the nauseating smells of her court. The queen's physician is said to have advised her that bathing was dangerous! Taking his advice, she had only one or two baths a year!

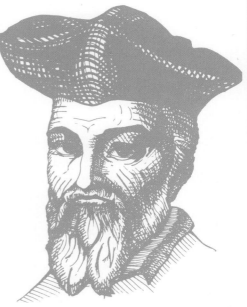

Nostradamus

During the sixteenth and seventeenth centuries in Renaissance Europe, the essential oils began to enjoy a resurgence. The perfumer's art was revived when Catherine de Medici, the queen of Henry II of France, created a fashion for aromatic products. Apparently, she adored the beautiful haunting fragrance of neroli, whose hypnotic, euphoric properties are known to act as an aphrodisiac, increasing sexual desire. Fascinated by the occult sciences, she regularly consulted Nostradamus, along with her court alchemist and astrologer. Catherine is said to have used the Dark Arts to dispatch a number of her enemies, using a few of the poisonous oils blended for this purpose by her court apothecaries!

By the end of the seventeenth century alchemy gave way to chemistry, and eventually the early nineteenth century saw the start of the scientific revolution. For the first time, chemists were able to identify the various properties of the essential oils, and as this research developed, it saw the development of synthetic chemicals. It is from these early beginnings that the modern drug industry developed. Natural medicines fell into decline. Gradually, health care became professionalized and individuals no longer treated themselves with natural remedies or folk medicine, but instead relied on medical doctors. These doctors were very expensive, so the poor still visited apothecaries.

Aromatherapy is a specialized branch of herbal medicine that consists of natural plant products and developed alongside herbalism, but both have a common root. The plants that yield the essential oils are also used in herbal medicine. In nineteenth-century Germany, books on distillation were beginning to appear, and it was at this time that the great European herbalists began to write their herbals, a number of which are still in print today. By the nineteenth century, with the advent of synthetic medicine, the practice of herbalism and the use of natural remedies and essential oils for therapeutic purposes faded out, as scientific medicine began to take over, and people began to place their faith in these new chemical drugs.

Eventually, with the rise of side effects and the realization that drugs were not the panacea they were once thought to be, the pendulum began to swing back to natural remedies and individual empowerment. People began to treat minor illnesses themselves, using the many natural medicines found in Mother Nature's pharmacy. Therapy through plants or the use of their aromatic essences using essential oils was an easy way to self-treat minor ailments, so modern aromatherapy began to take off.

The twentieth century saw the resurgence of essential oils used for therapeutic purposes. Rene Gattefosse, known as the Father of Aromatherapy, was the first to call this practice *aromatherapy*. His first book on the subject, titled *Aromatherapie*, was published in 1928. Following on was a medical doctor, Dr. Jean Valnet, who pioneered work with oils and published his findings in *The Practice of Aromatherapy*. Dr. Valnet had already enjoyed a long medical career when he began to use essential oils to treat infected wounds, burns, and gangrene during his work as a military surgeon in the Indochina rice fields on the front line at Tonkin. During this time, he noticed the beneficial effects of all

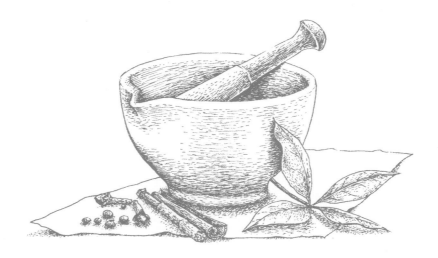

the constituent parts of whole plants, and he developed a profound interest in natural medicine. He also found these therapeutic plant oils to be successful in his work with psychiatric patients. This natural therapy was based on the use of whole plants, and Dr. Valnet was awarded numerous honorary distinctions for his work and experience in this field.

Two other pioneers who are credited with bringing aromatherapy back into the consciousness of the general public were Marguerite Maury, a biochemist who studied Dr. Valnet's work, and a name we have all heard of today, Robert Tisserand, whose book *The Art of Aromatherapy*, published in 1977, generated much interest and still does today. This age-old practice of natural health and beauty therapy has become very popular, and it is now tailored for use in a modern, stressful world. The beauty of essential oils is that they have multiple properties, and each oil has many uses. Let these mysterious oils, through regular use, enter your daily life to work their powerful alchemy!

❀ ❀ ❀

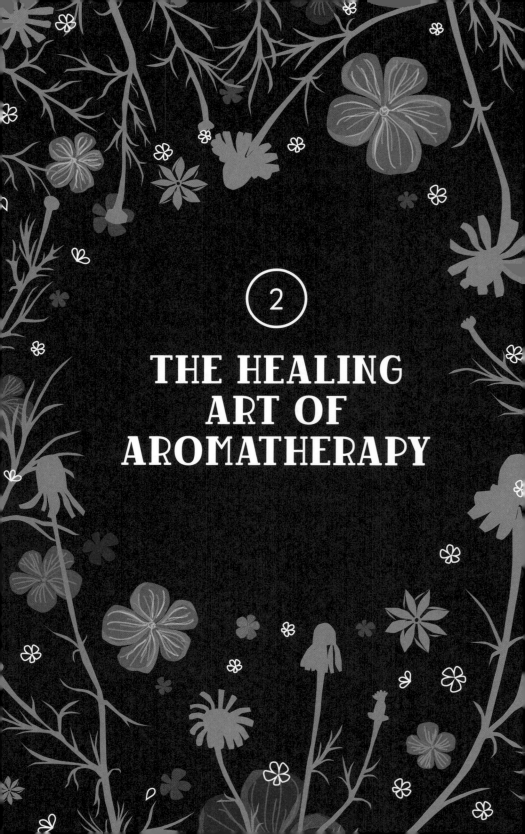

2

THE HEALING ART OF AROMATHERAPY

"There is a remedy for every illness to be found in nature."

Hippocrates

What Is an Essential Oil?

An essential oil is the pure concentrated substance found in selected aromatic plants. The essential oils are distilled from herbs, flowers, spices, fruits, trees, woods, and resins. These oils are the basis for aromatherapy treatments. The extracted oil has also been described as the plant's life force. The beneficial properties of pure essential oils are well known, and their status as natural, effective remedies with important physical and emotional benefits is widely accepted. Essential oils can be used in many different ways and for many different conditions. These very versatile oils are not used for just one purpose—they have multiple uses. You will find that many of the oils I mention in this book are used for a number of different conditions. Easy and pleasurable to use, each essential oil has its own aroma that falls into one of these fragrance families:

- floral
- spicy
- herbaceous
- green
- citrusy
- camphorous
- resinous
- earthy
- woody

You will find that because of their complex nature, most essential oils belong to more than one fragrance family and are therefore useful in a number of ways.

Each essential oil is made up of hundreds of different factors, and although these can be chemically identified, they have never been reproduced in a laboratory. Mother Nature's pharmacy is truly mysterious and has not yet yielded all of its secrets.

Professional aromatherapists today use about 300 essential oils, but these are not available to the general public. I will list the most popular oils that are publicly available (although some may be difficult to find) and details of their properties so that you can use them safely at home. When purchasing essential oils, always make sure they are from a good, reputable supplier—and, where possible, from wild-crafted sources—and the carrier oils cold-pressed so that only the highest-quality essential oils and base oils are extracted. Carrier oils are base oils, such as almond oil, into which a small amount of essential oil is dropped.

When it comes to these essential oils and the oils used for blending, you get what you pay for.

Patch Test

To check an oil, apply the diluted oil to a small patch of skin, on either the inner wrist or the inner elbow. Wait for an hour to check that there is no irritation or redness before using the oil.

Special Precautions

If you are asthmatic, pregnant, epileptic, have a skin condition, or are taking medications, it is suggested that before using any oil, you seek advice from a professional aromatherapist. Do not use essential oils on children without first consulting a professional aromatherapist.

How Oils Are Obtained

There are a number of different methods of extracting the oil from the raw material. Steam distillation and expression are the two most often used. Solvent extraction is also used.

Steam Distillation This is the most widely used method of producing the essential oil from the plant. A large still is filled with a quantity of the plant, covered with water, and steamed. The steam passes at high pressure through the plant material, releasing globules of essential oil into the water vapor. The fragrant steam is cooled back to water and the essential oil floats on the surface, which means it can be gently separated from the water and skimmed off. The lighter oils are seen floating on top and the heavier oils lying on the bottom.

Expression Citrus oils, which you've probably seen coming out of rinds when you've peeled fruit, are extracted using a method that involves pressing the oil directly out of the citrus fruit peel. Today this process is performed commercially by machines called centrifugal extractors.

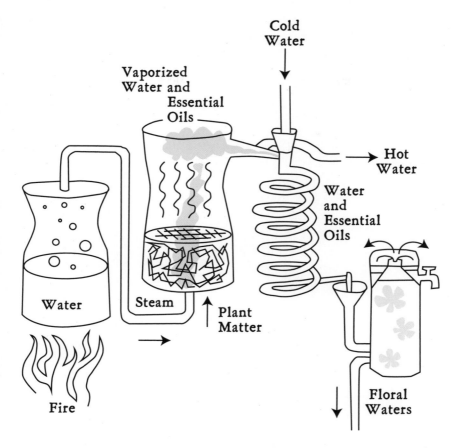

Solvent Extraction This method uses chemical solvents to dissolve the aromatic compounds out of delicate plant tissues in order to make "absolutes."

Absolute Oils Absolutes are highly aromatic liquids extracted from plants in a complex process. This requires the use of chemical solvents that are removed during the final stages of production. Absolutes are far more concentrated than regular essential oils, which is what makes them so special. Other methods of extraction do not extract much natural oil from the plant or harm the precious oil. They are much valued in aromatherapy, and they are used with care and respect. Absolutes are widely used in the perfume industry.

Safety Avoid using any essential oils therapeutically during pregnancy as they have not been scientifically validated for use by pregnant women.

✻ ✻ ✻

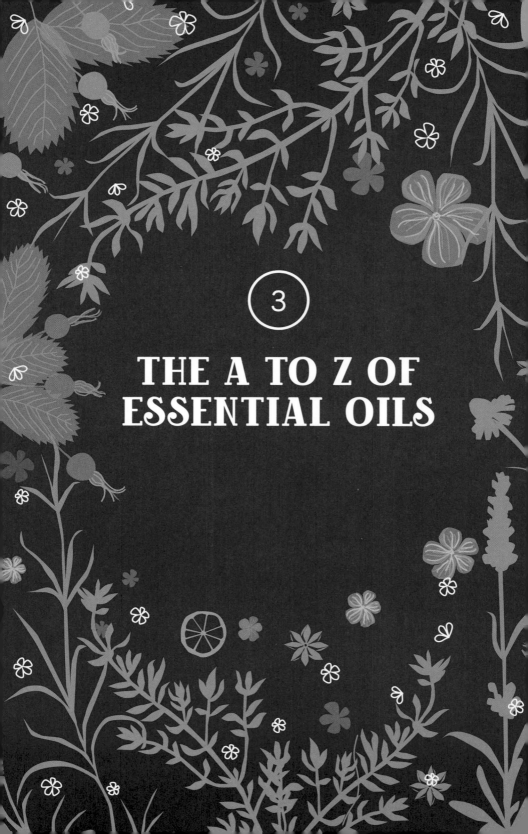

3

THE A TO Z OF ESSENTIAL OILS

"The Earth Laughs in Flowers."

Ralph Waldo Emerson

This chapter contains a concise dictionary of popular and useful essential oils, showing the original plant and, where appropriate, the exact part of the plant from which the oil comes. I then describe the kind of energy the oil provides, such as calming, energizing, and so on. I also offer information about the plant and suggest the best way to use it therapeutically. Where necessary, I mention any potential side effects.

Basil Oil

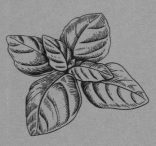

Parts used: flowering tops and leaves
Keywords: energizer and restorer
Aroma: herbaceous, fresh, and green

Description A delicate annual herb with dark green leaves and an uplifting, refreshing fragrance. Basil has been cultivated in Europe since the twelfth century. The name originated from the Greek meaning "king." Traditionally this herb has been used in Ayurveda, which is also known as the "Science of Life." This ancient Indian philosophy of health and well-being utilizes natural herbs, roots, plants, and essences in order to promote good health. In Ayurvedic medicine, basil is known as *tulsi*. Remains of basil oil have also been found in Egyptian burial chambers.

Uses Soothing, calming, and head-clearing. A therapeutic nerve tonic. Very popular as a culinary herb. Medicinally, basil's all-pervasive aroma is good for clearing the mind and aiding concentration, especially when tired. A focusing oil with a sweet, green refreshing smell, it relieves mental fatigue with its uplifting power.

Safety Not to be used pregnancy or for children.

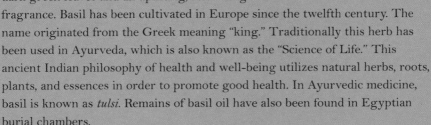

Bay Laurel Oil

Part used: tree and leaf
Keyword: uplifter
Aroma: bracing and pungent

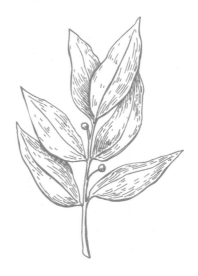

Description Bay laurels are tall
evergreen trees with glossy dark green
leaves and black berries. Traditionally the
leaves were used to weave a victorious
crown for Roman generals returning
from battle. "Laurels" were also used by
the Greeks for their returning heroes, as
a symbol of victory. Popular as a culinary
herb throughout Europe, the herb and oil
were also used medicinally for a variety of ailments.

Uses Mildly narcotic, bay laurel oil is still used by aromatherapists as a muscle
rub, for respiratory problems, and as a digestive. This oil may not be easily
available to the public due to its sedative properties, although it is still used in
scalp tonics on sale to the public.

Safety May cause skin irritation.

Benzoin Oil

Part used: tree resin
Keyword: decongestive
Aroma: sweet, rich, vanilla-like

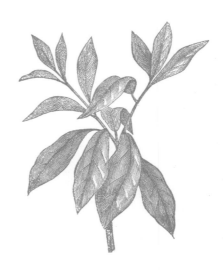

Description Distilled from the resin
of the Styrax tree, which grows in the
Far East. When the trunk is cut, a
balsamic, resinous sap exudes that has
a sweet, warm, vanilla-like smell. The
warm, relaxing scent of benzoin will

remind many of Friars Balsam, used as an inhalation for winter ills. Benzoin is a constituent of this inhalant. The essence is brown, thick, and sticky. Traditionally, it has been used for thousands of years in the East as incense and medicine.

Uses Used for the symptomatic relief of colds and sinusitis, benzoin has the ability to shift stubborn mucus. It also has sedative properties that relieve tension and stress.

Safety May cause irritation to sensitive skin.

Bergamot Oil

Part used: citrus rind (fruit peel)
Keyword: balancer
Aroma: delicious, sweet, citrusy

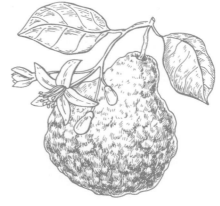

Description Made from a small tree with oval leaves bearing round, bitter, emerald-colored fruit resembling miniature oranges. Bergamot's deep green oil gives Earl Grey tea its distinctive aroma. This is one of the sweetest-smelling essential oils, released when the peels of the fruit are cold pressed. Traditionally, it has been used in Italian folk medicine for many years.

Uses This oil is restorative and can combat fatigue and stress. Bergamot's refreshing and relaxing properties help counteract low moods and uplift the spirits. It has deodorizing properties, too.

Safety Avoid if pregnant. May cause photosensitivity, so avoid using two to three hours before sunlight exposure.

Black Pepper Oil

Parts used: shrub and fruit
Keyword: warming tonic
Aroma: sharp, warming, spicy

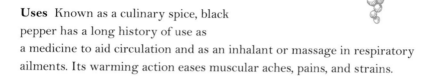

Description A perennial woody vine
with heart-shaped leaves. The berries
go from scarlet to black as they mature.
This oil has been used in the East
medicinally and for culinary purposes
for over 4,000 years.

Uses Known as a culinary spice, black
pepper has a long history of use as
a medicine to aid circulation and as an inhalant or massage in respiratory
ailments. Its warming action eases muscular aches, pains, and strains.

Safety May cause irritation to sensitive skin.

Cajuput Oil

Parts used: leaves, twigs, fresh buds of
the tree
Keyword: clearing
Aroma: strongly camphorous

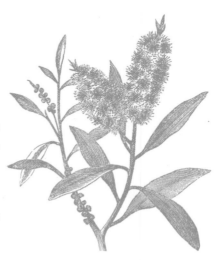

Description This Indonesian evergreen
tree is also known as the swamp tea tree.
It is a vigorous tree growing to about
45 feet (14 meters) high. The color of
the wood is white, and in Malaysia *caju-
puti* means "white wood," which is where
the name originates. Traditionally used
in the East in folk medicine for treating
many ailments as well as medicinally.

Uses Similar to eucalyptus due to its strong clear smell, cajuput oil is useful in inhalations and for respiratory support. It's an excellent choice for the winter months, due to its clearing properties.

Safety Nontoxic but may cause skin irritation in high concentrations.

Cedarwood Oil (Virginian)

Part used: tree/wood
Keyword: tranquilizer
Aroma: harmonious, earthy, woody

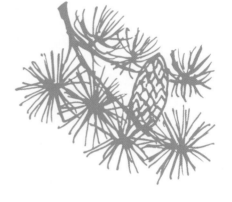

Description This slow-growing coniferous evergreen tree grows to great heights and can reach 120 feet (37 meters). Traditionally cedarwood was used by the Native Americans medicinally for respiratory infections and catarrhal conditions. It was used by many cultures for religious and purification rituals. The ancient Egyptians used this precious oil for embalming the dead.

Uses Cedarwood has a calming effect with a mild, sweet, woody aroma. It is also fortifying and strengthening. This oil's warm and dry properties are helpful in many skin conditions, particularly oily and problem skin, due to its astringent qualities. It is also a good expectorant and has sedative powers.

Safety May cause irritation to sensitive skin.

Chamomile Oil (Roman)

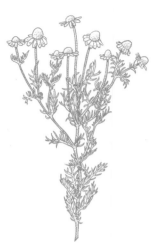

Parts used: dried flowers/buds
Keyword: strong-soother
Aroma: earthy, herbaceous, apple-like

Description A trailing perennial herb with
feathery leaves and daisy-like white flowers.
Traditionally, the ancient Egyptians used
this herb to cure fevers (heat) and dedicated it
to the Sun. Chamomile has been used in the
Mediterranean region for over 2,000 years.

Uses This versatile oil has many useful
qualities and can be used to treat a wide range of conditions. It is an excellent
oil to use for all types of skin care, especially sensitive and problematic skin.

Safety May cause dermatitis in some individuals.

Cinnamon Oil

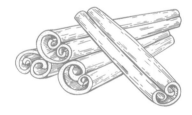

Part used: leaf
Keyword: antiseptic-tonic
Aroma: warm, spicy with
sweet undertones

Description A tropical evergreen
tree with green leathery leaves that have a spicy smell when bruised. The bark
is highly aromatic. Traditionally cinnamon oil has been used in the East for
thousands of years to treat a wide range of health complaints.

Uses Cinnamon leaf oil has antiseptic properties and exerts a therapeutic effect
on the immune and circulatory systems. It treats chills and poor circulation and
is supportive during outbreaks of colds and flu. The bark oil is not used, as it is
highly irritating to skin and mucous membranes.

Safety May be irritating to sensitive skin.

Citronella Oil

Part used: leaves and stems
Keyword: bug-buster
Aroma: sharp, lemony

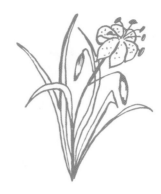

Description A tall perennial grass growing wild in Sri Lanka. Traditionally the leaves have been used by many cultures for their medicinal value.

Uses This essential oil is an excellent flying-insect repellent. It has a lemony aroma that insects hate. It also has powerful deodorant and antiseptic powers and is used as a stimulant and tonic. Good for deodorizing and vaporing.

Safety May be irritating to sensitive skin.

Clary Sage Oil

Parts used: flowering tops and foliage
Keyword: euphoric
Aroma: warm, nutty, and green

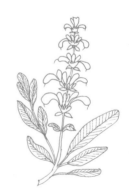

Description This plant is said to be native to Spain, but it is also found in the United States. When fully grown this shrubby herb reaches about 2 feet (61 cm) high. It has large purple flowers with leaves that smell of pineapple. It is associated with feminine sexuality. Traditionally the herb was once used for clearing mucus from the eyes. Today it is often found in perfumes.

Uses This oil is a muscle relaxant that helps in relieving pain. It is also used as a tonic for the female reproductive system and for treating menstrual problems, bringing back balance at certain times of the month.

Safety No known problems, but dilute well anyway.

Cypress Oil

Parts used: tree, leaves, cones
Keyword: woody-antiseptic
Aroma: woody and spicy

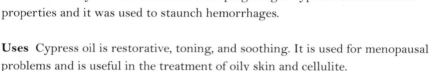

Description This tall evergreen tree is a familiar feature in Greek cemeteries. The wood is reddish-yellow in color with brown-gray cones. Traditionally, cypress has been associated with death, so the ancient Greeks and Romans planted it in their burial grounds. It was once used medicinally to treat childhood whooping cough. Cypress has hemostatic properties and it was used to staunch hemorrhages.

Uses Cypress oil is restorative, toning, and soothing. It is used for menopausal problems and is useful in the treatment of oily skin and cellulite.

Safety Not usually problematic, but dilute well.

Eucalyptus Oil (Globulus)

Parts used: tree and leaves
Keyword: easy-breather
Aroma: fresh, green, medicinal, camphorous

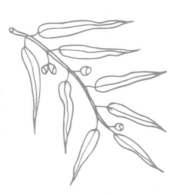

Description This tall evergreen tree, native to Tasmania and Australia, reaches a great height. Traditionally a household remedy made with this oil from the Australian gum-tree was used for respiratory problems, and it still is today.

Uses This well-known camphorous oil has strong antibacterial properties. It is used as a decongestant and expectorant in colds and chest infections and is a useful oil for inhalations.

Safety Do not ingest or use if you have epilepsy.

Frankincense Oil

Part used: tree/bark
Keyword: rejuvenator
Aroma: spicy, woody, and balsamic

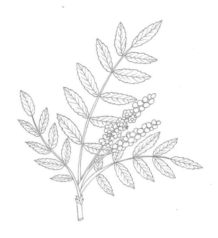

Description A small tree or shrub that yields gum resin from the bark, where the oil is found. This valuable oil is native to Somalia. Traditionally, frankincense was used in ancient Egypt for cosmetic purposes, and it has also been used in India, China, and the West as an incense, and medicinally in the East.

Uses This wonderful oil has a wide range of properties. In the West it is recognized as an excellent anti-ageing oil for mature skin. Known for its rejuvenating and toning effect, this beauty oil can be used in anti-ageing face creams or blended with other anti-ageing oils. Medicinally, frankincense is used for chest problems, coughs, and colds. Its calming properties can help treat anxiety, tension, and stress.

Safety No currently known precautions.

Geranium Oil

Parts used: flowers and leaves
Keyword: hormone-balancer
Aroma: floral, sweet, heavy

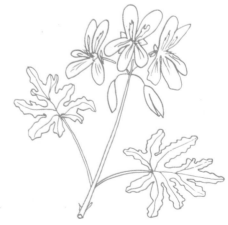

Description An attractive, strongly scented perennial shrub with serrated, pointed leaves and small flowers. There are a large number of different types of geranium flowers, but only seven of them are used to make the oil.

Harvesting takes place when the flowers start to bloom. Traditionally this plant used to be grown around cottages to keep evil spirits away. Medicinally it was regarded as a healing plant used for treating wounds and tumors and for protection against insect bites.

Uses This oil appears to exert a regulatory function on the female hormonal system and is useful for premenstrual tension and menopausal problems. Its astringent qualities make it good for all skin types. Its analgesic properties help ease the pain of shingles and neuralgia.

Safety Safe oil but may cause irritation to sensitive skin.

Grapefruit Oil

Parts used: tree and citrus rind (fruit peel)
Keyword: energizer
Aroma: sharp, citrusy, and refreshing

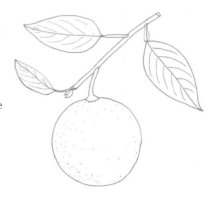

Description A tree with glossy leaves. The oil glands buried deep within the peel yield only a small amount of oil. Traditionally originating in tropical Asia and the West Indies, the tree is now mainly cultivated in North and South America.

Uses This oil is helpful in the treatment of oily skin, supports the liver, and helps cleanse the lymphatic system. Colds and flu with hot, feverish symptoms respond well to its cooling, antiseptic qualities that help loosen mucus and catarrh.

Safety May cause photosensitivity, so do not use two to three hours before sunlight exposure.

Jasmine Oil

Parts used: tree and flowers
Keyword: relaxant
Aroma: sweet, heady, and exotic

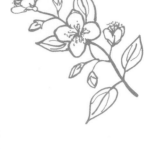

Description This oil is known as the "King of Flowers." It originates from Iran and northern India. Jasmine is a highly valued oil in perfumery, but it has many more properties than just a beautiful, uplifting aroma. In times past, it was used in love potions as well as in the treatment of venereal diseases.

Uses Jasmine's refreshing and soothing actions help relax tense muscles and feelings of tightness in the chest area. Its aphrodisiac properties are well known, and this oil is used for enjoyment and pleasure and for the sheer beauty of the exotic aroma. Jasmine can be used as a natural perfume applied undiluted on the pulse points.

Safety No known toxicity.

Juniper Berry Oil

Parts used: bush and berries
Keyword: toxin-eliminator
Aroma: fresh yet woody and balsamic

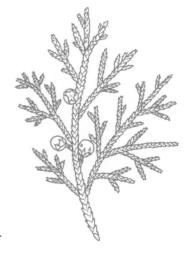

Description This evergreen coniferous shrub has needle-like leaves and fleshy berries that turn blue-black with a white bloom during the second year of growth. It grows in many regions of the world. Juniper berries are what gives gin its unique flavor. Traditionally, juniper oil was used to help combat contagious diseases such as typhoid and cholera. In Tibetan medicine, it was used to help prevent the plague. In ancient Greece and Rome and in Arabia, its antiseptic properties were valued.

Uses An uplifting and purifying oil, juniper is a good detoxifier and immune booster, helping to prevent illness. It is an antiseptic tonic, making it ideal for use on greasy, congested skin, and its purifying properties help many skin disorders.

Safety Avoid if you have any type of kidney disorder.

Lavender Oil

Parts used: leaves, flowers, and buds
Keyword: balancer
Aroma: light, floral

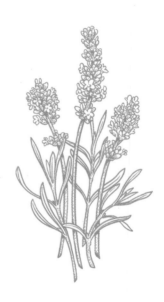

Description This attractive evergreen perennial plant has intensely fragrant blue-mauve flowers, and it is extensively cultivated in England and France. It is the most versatile, classic, and beautifully scented of all healing oils and has been widely used for centuries. The Romans used this antiseptic oil for bathing and to cleanse lacerations and wounds after battle. The name itself originates from the Latin *lavare*, which means "to wash."

Uses An amazing oil with many benefits and uses, lavender can be helpful in a number of conditions and situations. It is used to promote relaxation and a good night's sleep and is a useful first-aid remedy for all sorts of skin problems. Lavender has mild analgesic properties and many applications to health.

Safety Use with care if you have low blood pressure.

Lemon

Parts used: fruit and citrus rind (fruit peel)
Keyword: stimulator
Aroma: sharp, fresh, and cleansing

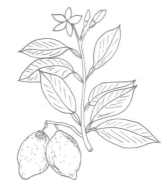

Description A thorny evergreen tree that is native to India. Because of its antiseptic qualities, lemon was used to treat malaria and to guard against bites from disease-carrying insects. The Crusaders brought the lemon fruit back to Europe on their return from the Middle East.

Uses Lemon is useful for boosting sluggish circulation and clarifying greasy skin and as a lymphatic cleanser. Its diuretic qualities are useful in reducing cellulite. Lemon stimulates the immune system, helping to prevent colds and ward off infections.

Lemongrass Oil

Parts used: grass and leaves
Keyword: antiseptic-toner
Aroma: sweet and lemony

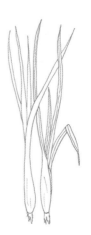

Description This oil is produced by steam distillation from two species of fresh lemongrass, namely, West Indian and East Indian. Both have similar qualities. Lemongrass originated in tropical Asia, and it is cultivated in India, Sri Lanka, Indonesia, Africa, and Madagascar. It was thought to be helpful in bringing down fevers.

Uses Lemongrass oil is very antiseptic and is useful in protecting against airborne infections. It is uplifting and a good tonic, with mild antidepressant properties. Its pain-relieving properties are useful for treating sore or strained muscles, especially after sports.

Safety Nontoxic but avoid if skin is sensitive or damaged.

Mandarin Oil

Parts used: tree and citrus rind (fruit peel)
Keyword: childhood-soother
Aroma: sweet, tangy

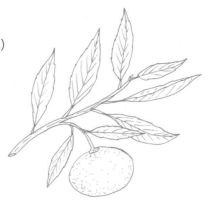

Description A small evergreen tree with dark green shiny leaves and fragrant flowers that ripen into fruit. This oil was traditionally used in France to strengthen the digestive function. It is still used for that purpose. This citrus fruit has associations with Christmas.

Uses Mandarin is an antispasmodic and nervous sedative that has a soothing effect on digestive problems, dyspepsia, and constipation. This oil is well liked for use with restless and hyperactive children due to its soothing, calming effect. Mandarin's aroma is delicate and sweet, unlike the stronger, zestier citrus oils.

Safety May cause photosensitivity, so do not use two to three hours before sunlight exposure.

Marjoram Oil

Parts used: flowering heads and leaves
Keyword: comforter
Aroma: sweet, green, herbaceous

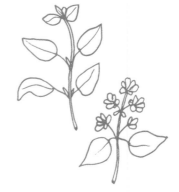

Description A bushy perennial herb that is strongly aromatic. Sweet marjoram originates in North Africa, Egypt, and the Mediterranean regions. The sweet, sticky resin this herb secretes is popular with bees. Traditionally it was used for culinary purposes and as a folk remedy. The ancient Greeks used marjoram oil in cosmetics, perfumes, and medicines.

Uses Warm and comforting, this oil is useful for aching muscles and lower back pain. Marjoram's antispasmodic properties are useful in treating digestive problems. This is a good oil to blend with other warming oils such as rosemary to soothe tired, aching muscles.

Safety Nontoxic in dilution.

Melissa Oil

Parts used: flowers and leaves
Keyword: hormone-balancer (female)
Aroma: herby, lemony, with sweet undertones

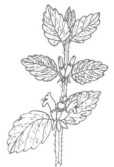

Description Also known as lemon balm, the yellowish flowers attract bees, hence the name *Melissa*, which is the Greek word for "bee." A Mediterranean plant, it grows to about 2 feet (61 cm) high. Most of the oil is produced in France. Introduced into Britain by the Romans, it was used by French Carmelite nuns in the fourteenth century to make tonic water. During the Elizabethan Age, the leaves were used in wine making. Today, products labeled as melissa oil are usually a blend of citrus oils because the pure oil is very expensive.

Uses Melissa oil is helpful in reducing anxiety and relieving headaches associated with neck and shoulder pain and tension. Inflamed skin conditions and eczema benefit from this oil, especially when the condition is stress-related. It has a mild antihistamine action that is helpful for hay-fever sufferers.

Safety May cause irritation to sensitive skin.

Myrrh Oil

Part used: resin
Keyword: strengthening-healer
Aroma: earthy, warm, woody, balsamic

Description This well-known shrub is a native of
North Africa. It grows to about 9 feet (3 meters)
high and when the gray bark is cut, the gum resin
exudes. It is from this slightly musky-smelling resin
that the oil is distilled. Traditionally, its use was widespread in the ancient
world. It had a broad medicinal use among the ancient Egyptians, and it was
used in mummification as well as in cosmetics. Greek soldiers took a phial of
myrrh to battle, as it helped stem bleeding wounds due to its anti-inflammatory
and antiseptic properties.

Uses This oil is an excellent expectorant when there is thick mucus. It is
useful in treating digestive ailments and in dental health and skin care.

Safety Nonirritant in dilution. Do not use in high concentrations.

Myrtle Oil

Parts used: leaves
Keyword: regulator
Aroma: sweet and penetrating

Description This small evergreen tree with blue-green
leaves grows throughout the Mediterranean. It was
traditionally used medicinally by the ancient Egyptians
and the Romans. Famed as an aphrodisiac, myrtle oil was added to love potions.

Uses It is used for respiratory disorders due to its sedative qualities and for
genito-urinary problems in men and women. Not always easily available for
public use.

Safety Prolonged use can irritate mucous membranes.

Neroli Oil

Part used: orange tree blossoms
Keyword: de-stressor
Aroma: sensual floral, with a balancing effect

Description This orange tree originally came
from China. The expensive essential oil is
extracted from the flowers of the bitter Seville
orange, which is at home in a Mediterranean or
subtropical climate. Orange flower petals, symbolizing innocence and purity,
were used in wedding bouquets. The petals were also used to make *eau de
cologne* for Victorian ladies when they had the "vapors." The "vapors" were
either genuinely stress-related responses to shock, or hysterics that were put on
for dramatic effect.

Uses This stress-reliever is useful for hormonal and menopausal disorders.
Relaxing and uplifting, neroli is an excellent oil to use on skin that has begun
to wrinkle and develop broken capillaries.

Safety No known precautions.

Niaouli

Parts used: tree, shoots, twigs, leaves
Keyword: clearing
Aroma: sweetly penetrating and antiseptic

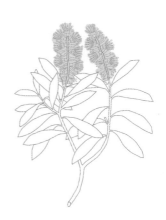

Description Related to the tea tree, this
evergreen tree's leaves exude a strong antiseptic,
medicinal aroma when crushed. Niaouli has
been used for a wide variety of ailments and
also for purifying water. It is used by French
obstetricians because of its strong antiseptic
actions.

Uses This immune-system booster promotes antibody activity that helps fight infections. It is good to use for respiratory problems and may also be effective in helping to clear urinary tract infections.

Safety No problems have been reported, but a patch test is still recommended.

Orange Oil

Parts used: fruit and peel
Keyword: detoxifier
Aroma: refreshing, zesty citrus scent

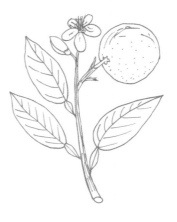

Description This oil is extracted from the fruits and peels of certain citrus trees, and it has tranquilizing, soothing, and calming properties. The orange tree has also given us neroli from the orange blossoms, and petitgrain from the leaves and twigs of this lovely citrus tree. Today it is found growing abundantly in the Mediterranean region. In Chinese medicine, the dried sweet orange peel has been used to treat a number of ailments, namely, coughs, colds, anorexia, and breast sores.

Uses This oil is a favorite addition to baths during winter and is helpful for those having trouble getting to sleep. It is a good detoxifier and cleanser that supports the lymphatic system.

Safety May cause photosensitivity. May cause irritation to sensitive skin.

Palmarosa Oil

Parts used: grass and leaves
Keyword: balancer
Aroma: sweet rosy and floral

Description A wild-growing herbaceous plant native
to India and Pakistan. The grassy-smelling leaves
have a strong fragrance. Traditionally this oil dates back to a time when it
was transported to ports of the Red Sea from Bombay and brought by land to
Bulgaria and Constantinople, now known as Istanbul.

Uses This is a strengthening oil for the nervous system and for skin support.
It has antiviral properties, is cooling and toning, and has balancing actions that
make it useful in treating stress, anxiety, and tension.

Safety No currently known precautions. Use in dilution.

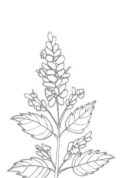

Patchouli Oil

Part used: leaves
Keyword: strengthener
Aroma: earthy, heavy, persistent, woody

Description This perennial bushy herb is found
in the Far East and grows up to about three feet
(one meter) high. Its large, fragrant leaves exude
an exotic scent reminiscent of India. Traditionally, patchouli oil was used in
the East to scent linen. Believed to prevent disease, it was used medicinally in
China, Malaysia, and Japan as an antidote to insect and snake bites.

Uses Patchouli oil is useful in treating inflamed skin conditions, acne, and
greasy skin. Its antidepressant actions are helpful in the treatment of anxious
and stressful conditions. This oil's relaxing qualities make it good for use
during meditation. Antiseptic, antidepressant, and aphrodisiac.

Safety No currently known precautions. Use in dilution.

Peppermint Oil

Parts used: herb leaves and flowering tops
Keyword: refresher
Aroma: invigorating, green, and minty

Description Native to Europe, this plant likes to grow
in damp conditions, and its high-reaching stem grows
to about 3 feet (1 meter). This herb was known to
the ancient Egyptians, Greeks, and Romans. It was used in Roman feasts and
celebrations to calm the digestion of Romans who had eaten too much after
their revelries. Peppermint has stimulating and uplifting properties.

Uses Because of its head-clearing action, peppermint is used for headaches,
migraines, and insomnia. It can give relief from painful digestive spasms and
bloating, so it is a well-known therapeutic treatment for irritable bowel syndrome.

Safety Care should be taken with the dosage, due to its powerful aroma, and it
can be problematic for anyone with heart ailments. Use in dilution.

Petitgrain

Parts used: leaves and twigs of the orange tree
Keyword: stimulant
Aroma: woody, haunting, citrusy

Description The oil is extracted from the twigs
and leaves of the orange tree. The best-quality oil
comes from France. The leaves were once used in
the treatment of epilepsy.

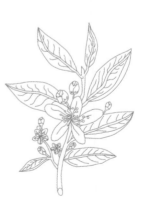

Uses Petitgrain oil has a vibrant citrus aroma
and it is a natural deodorant. It has antidepressant
and sedative properties that make it useful in treating ailments of the nervous
system. Added to a final hair rinse, this oil can encourage healthy hair growth.

Safety No currently known cautions. Use in dilution.

Pine Oil

Parts used: tree needles and cones
Keyword: cleanser
Aroma: piercing and refreshing forest

Description There are about eighty species of this
large conifer. Much of the oil is obtained from the
species of Scots and Norwegian pine. Many ancient
civilizations used it medicinally, due to its curative and cleansing properties, to
treat respiratory infections. Pine oil is also associated with religious ceremonies.

Uses Strongly antiseptic, this cleansing and clearing oil is effective in
inhalations. It protects against bacterial and viral infections, clears stubborn
catarrh, and helps alleviate sinus infections. Its bracing and fortifying aroma
can lift mental fatigue and calm nervous tension.

Safety May cause irritation to sensitive skin. Avoid strong concentrations—so
restrict to less than 2 percent in a carrier oil, such as almond oil.

Ravensara Oil

Part used: leafy twigs
Keyword: pain-reliever
Aroma: warm, camphorous

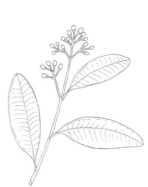

Description Produced in Madagascar, the oil is
steam distilled from young, leafy twigs. Every part
of the tree is aromatic. It is traditionally used as
a tonic, and medicinally for all kinds of infectious conditions. The word itself
originates from a Malagasy phrase that means "the leaf is good for you."

Uses This warm, stimulating oil acts on the mind and on emotional issues.
It also helps the respiratory and digestive systems, and its pain-relieving
properties are helpful in rheumatic and arthritic conditions.

Safety Safe in dilution.

Rose Otto Oil

Parts used: flower and petals
Keyword: heaven-scent
Aroma: warm and floral

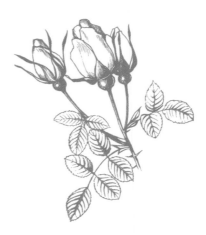

Description Rose otto is the "queen" of all essential oils. This small prickly shrub has beautiful blooms with a very strong fragrance, and it grows prolifically. Originating in Persia, this is an enhancing oil known to bring physical and emotional stability. Persian soldiers going into battle adorned their shields with a red rose. During the Middle Ages, this oil was used to cool inflammation. Rose otto is one of the finest essential oils but it is extremely expensive. It is known to prevent skin damage. Damask rose is the variety most often used in aromatherapy.

Uses Rose otto is helpful on dry skin, broken capillaries, and mature and sensitive complexions. Depression, headaches, and nervous tension also benefit from this lovely rose oil. It has a clearing effect on the female reproductive system.

Safety Nontoxic. Safe in dilution.

Rosemary Oil

Parts used: herb flowering tops and leaves
Keyword: restorer
Aroma: fresh and green

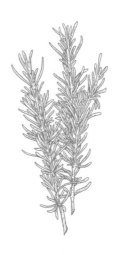

Description An evergreen with needle-shaped leaves. Bees love its bluish lilac flowers. Traditionally, ancient civilizations regarded the rosemary bush as sacred and used it for medicine and food and in magical ceremonies.

Uses A piercing scent makes rosemary oil useful for inhalations. It aids memory and concentration, and it can also combat fatigue. This oil is used for treating women's health problems related to painful periods, respiratory infections, and afflictions of the nervous system.

Safety Avoid if you have high blood pressure or epilepsy. Safe in dilution.

Rosewood Oil

Parts used: tree/wood
Keyword: balancer
Aroma: sweet, woody, and musky

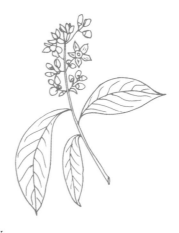

Description This tall evergreen tree grows in the lush tropical rain forests of Brazil. The oil is distilled from the heartwood of the tree. The rose-scented wood was used to make furniture in France. The oil has been used in the perfumery industry, but rosewood oil has only been recently introduced into aromatherapy.

Uses Rosewood oil aids the respiratory system and is useful in treating stress-related conditions. It is recommended for balancing the emotions. This oil relieves headaches associated with nausea, stabilizes the central nervous system, and boosts an underfunctioning immune system

Safety No currently known precautions. Safe in dilution.

Sandalwood Oil

Parts used: bark and inner heartwood
Keyword: relaxer
Aroma: sweet, lingering, and exotic

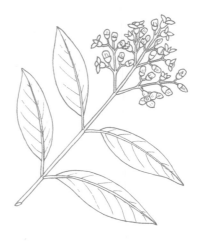

Description Originating in southern
Asia, this oil is an important therapy
in traditional Chinese medicine and
Ayurvedic medicine. The oil is distilled
from the heartwood of the tree.
Traditionally this oil is mentioned in
Old Sanskrit and Chinese manuscripts.
Many deities and temples were carved
from this aromatic wood, and the oil was used in religious ritual.

Uses Sandalwood oil is used as a massage oil and it is useful for dry and
allergic skin. Its cooling properties can soothe inflamed mucous membranes in
respiratory ailments. It is said to have aphrodisiac properties that are reputed
to increase the male libido. Genito-urinary tract infections can be treated with
sandalwood. Its antiseptic properties can clear pus and infections.

Safety Safe in dilution, but avoid if you have depression.

Tea Tree Oil

Part used: leaves
Keyword: first aider
Aroma: medicinal, woody, and earthy

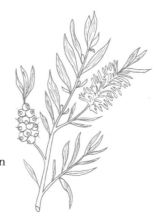

Description Originating in New South Wales,
Australia, this colorless, strong antiseptic oil
smells very medicinal. Crushed leaves were used
by the aborigines to treat infected wounds and skin
problems, but it was only after the First World
War that anyone gave serious thought to its use.

Before antibiotics came into existence, soldiers on the battlefields were treated with tea tree oil, which was kept in first-aid kits. Though relatively unknown outside Australia for many years, it is now a major force for healing.

Uses An excellent germicidal and fungicidal agent against virulent organisms. Tea tree is a bacteriostat; this means that it stops bacterial growth, so it is valuable today when bacteria are becoming resistant to many antibiotics. This oil is also a great all-purpose cleaner.

Safety Nontoxic externally, but may cause irritation to sensitive skin.

Thyme

Parts used: flowers and leaves
Keyword: bacterial-cleanser
Aroma: fresh, green, and herbaceous

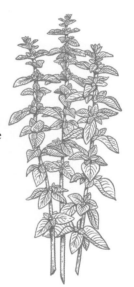

Description Native to Europe, particularly around the Mediterranean, thyme has now spread all over the world. It is thought to have been used as long ago as 3,500 BCE by the Sumerians. The ancient Egyptians used it for embalming, while the Greeks used it for medicinal purposes, and they still do. It was also used by the Romans for cookery and medicinally. Until the First World War, thyme oil was used with clove, lemon, and chamomile as a disinfectant in hospitals.

Uses Thyme is useful in warm baths and as a rub for joint pains, backache, and sciatica. It boosts immunity by stimulating the white blood cells, enabling them to fight off infections. Muscles and joints also benefit from thyme oil's therapeutic actions that ease stiffness and arthritic conditions.

Safety Avoid sensitive or damaged skin. Do a patch test. Use well diluted and avoid if you have high blood pressure. In baths, dilute thyme oil below 1 percent. Prolonged use can cause toxicity.

Vanilla

Part used: resinoid from vanilla beans
Keyword: uplifter
Aroma: rich, sweet, and balsamic

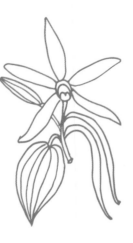

Description This perennial climbing vine produces green capsules of fruit and is known as a balsamic resinoid. Traditionally, when the plant is grown it has to be hand-pollinated, but in Mexico, the hummingbirds do this instead!

Uses Vanilla is used as a fragrance in Oriental perfumes and pharmaceutical products. In aromatherapy, it is used only for use in burners and diffusers.

Safety Do not use medicinally for massage or skin care.

Vetiver

Parts used: grass and root
Keyword: tranquilizer
Aroma: smoky, woody, earthy

Description Vetiver is a wild tall perennial grass found in tropical areas. It is cultivated in the tropical and subtropical climates of Asia. The oil is distilled from the rootlets. The older root produces the better oil. Vetiver is known as the oil of tranquility due to its sedating and calming action.

Uses Its sedating and strengthening action makes it ideal for use in massages and baths. It is also useful in the treatment of acne and other skin problems. Vetiver eases liver congestion, stimulates circulation, and eases muscular pain. It is supportive when one is feeling emotionally low.

Safety Safe in dilution. No currently known precautions.

Ylang-Ylang Oil

Part used: leaves, flowers, buds
Keyword: lover's enjoyment
Aroma: heavy, exotic, sensual/floral

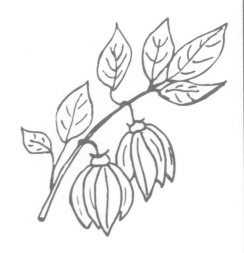

Description Ylang-ylang originates
in the Philippines and has now spread
throughout tropical Asia. It was used
as an ingredient of hair preparations in
Europe, and the name means "flower of
flowers." The oil has been used in folk
medicine in the Far East and in skin
creams, helping keep skin hydrated and
young looking.

Uses This oil is useful for treating low blood pressure and nervous or
emotional palpitations. It helps relax the mind and emotions, and balances
blood pressure and a rapid heartbeat. Ylang-ylang's calming action creates a
sense of well-being, and its aphrodisiac properties relax inhibitions for both
men and women. It relaxes and arouses at the same time, due to its amazing
adaptogenic properties.

Safety The strong odor may cause headaches. Do not use with inflammatory
skin conditions. It may cause irritation on sensitive skin. Use well diluted.

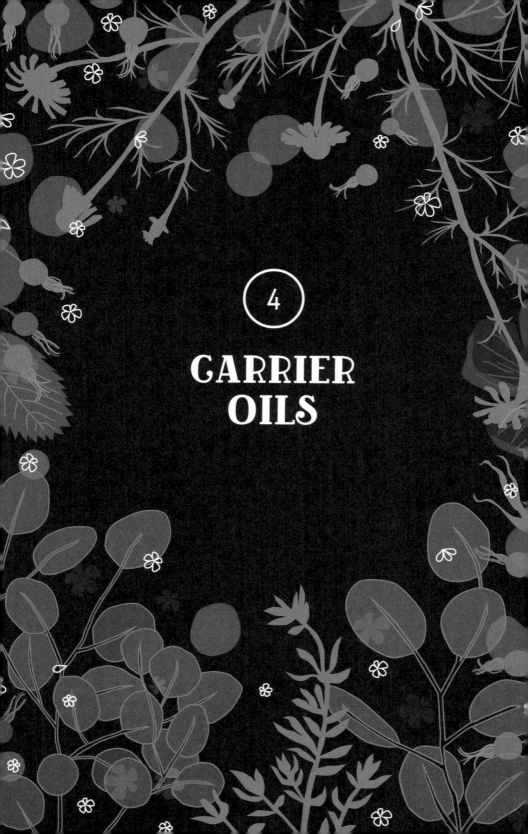

4

CARRIER
OILS

Essential oils are powerful, concentrated substances and almost all must be diluted in a carrier oil before use. Carrier oils are facilitators that allow the essential oils to work their magic. These base oils used to dilute aromatherapy oils come from nuts, seeds, and vegetables. They are easily absorbed by the skin, and it is important to use an unrefined, good-quality carrier oil in order to gain the full therapeutic benefit. Before use, it is best to do a patch test to see if you react in any way. There are a number of these carrier oils, and some will be suitable for home use. I recommend that you have a whole range of these therapeutic oils in your beauty toolkit, as they have beneficial properties of their own. Try to buy cold-pressed oils, as these will have retained all the vitamins, minerals, and fatty acids.

Almond Oil

Sweet almond oil is one of the most popular carrier oils. It is a light, odorless oil that is ideal as a face and body massage oil. Rich in vitamins, minerals, and protein, it can be used on all types of skin, but it is particularly beneficial for dry and problem skin. Cold-pressed almond oil is ideal to use as a massage base and also in the bath.

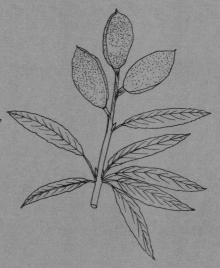

Apricot-Kernel Oil

This light-textured oil is extracted from the stones of the fruit, and it is especially suitable for dry, mature skin, but it can work on all skin types. It improves elasticity and is an ideal carrier oil to use as a base for facial massage blends. Rich in vitamins and minerals, it can be blended with less expensive oils such as grapeseed, almond, or jojoba.

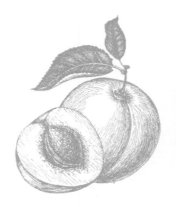

Argan Oil

This soothing and moisturizing plant oil is high in omega fatty acids and vitamin E. It is produced from the kernel of the argan tree that grows abundantly in Morocco. Argan oil has become popular and is easy to obtain in health shops. It is an ideal base oil that supports the skin's overall health. Nongreasy and nonirritating, argan is useful for healing and hydrating the skin, giving it a healthy boost.

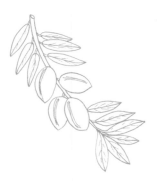

Avocado Oil

This rich, green, heavy, viscous oil contains vitamins A and E and is an amazing conditioner for dry, dehydrated, and mature skin. The vitamin E content of this oil is vital for skin health. This important beauty vitamin is known as an antioxidant. Antioxidants help fight off the damaging free radicals that age the skin prematurely. Avocado oil has another remarkable property: it is anti-inflammatory, so is an excellent oil to use for healing sun-damaged skin. Too heavy to use on its own, this oil is best blended with any of the basic carrier oils.

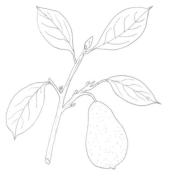

Evening Primrose Oil

This fabulous oil was used by Native American
medicine men who knew of its therapeutic
properties for wound healing. EPO is good
for older complexions, due to its very rich
content of GLA (gamma linolenic acid) and
vitamins. A precious ingredient, GLA helps to
combat dry, devitalized skin. EPO oil is a star
in natural medicine, and it is also very popular
for internal use. This oil may, with regular
use, externally help to prevent premature skin
ageing, support regeneration, and protect against moisture loss. Taking the oil
internally in the form of capsules can also improve the skin's appearance. Due
to its heavy, viscous consistency, EPO is best added to a basic carrier oil.

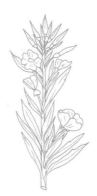

Grapeseed Oil

This oil, extracted from grape pips, is a favorite with
aromatherapists due to its light texture and easy
absorption. Because it has the least odor of all the oils,
it allows the fragrance of the essential oils that will
be used with it to come through. It is ideal for general
body massage, as it does not leave a greasy feeling on
the skin. Grapeseed oil is not particularly nourishing,
though, so it benefits from the addition of richer oils in various blends, but this
depends on what it is to be used for.

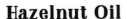

Hazelnut Oil

This pale-yellow oil contains anti-ageing, nourishing,
and antioxidant properties. It is extremely light and
is good for oily and combination skins due to its
astringent properties.

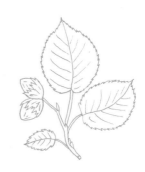

Jojoba Oil

This base oil has a long history of use among
Native Americans. It is actually a liquid wax and
therefore an excellent carrier oil for use with
essential oils. Golden yellow in color, jojoba is an
excellent softening and moisturizing oil. It is light,
nongreasy, and a good base when making up facial
blends, as it is easily absorbed due to the fact that
it resembles the skin's own natural oils. Versatile, it
can be used for facial massage and also for body and
hair care. Every skin type can benefit from the use of this "liquid gold."

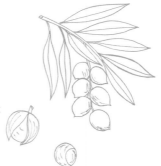

Macadamia Oil

Rich in vitamins and essential fatty acids, this oil
has a fine texture and is good in blends used for
skin care. It is especially beneficial for mature and
ageing skin. Virgin cold-pressed is best to use, but
it is not easy to find on sale to the public. If you
want to use macadamia oil, you must find a good-
quality essential oil supplier.

Peach-Kernel Oil

This oil comes from the nut of the peach fruit.
It is lighter than sweet almond oil and is good
for dry, ageing skin that has thread veins. Fine
textured, it is easily absorbed and rich in vitamin
E—a powerful antioxidant—and essential
fatty acids. This oil is also suitable for sensitive
complexions. Easily absorbed, it is ideal to use as a massage base.

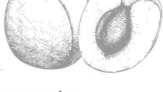

Rosehip Oil

This rejuvenating oil has traditionally been used for hundreds of years in South American countries for its healing properties. Rosehip oil has been shown to heal burns, scars, and stretch marks. Used in blends for skin regeneration, its rich, hydrating, essential fatty acid content includes omegas 3 and 6 in the form of GLA (gamma linolenic acid). The oil encourages tissue repair. Due to its high fat content, rosehip oil is very good for use in prematurely ageing skin, helping to improve skin radiance when skin is lackluster. This magical oil has also been found to smooth away wrinkles and crow's feet.

Wheatgerm Oil

The ancient Egyptians used this oil, and it has been found in tombs dating back 2,000 years. Highly nourishing, rich, and aromatic, wheatgerm oil is extracted from the wheatgerm that contains the life force of the plant. If unrefined, it is rich in vitamin E, the beauty vitamin, and its powerful antioxidant properties heal scar tissue, burns, and stretch marks. Wheatgerm oil's consistency is too sticky to use alone as it is the heaviest of the carrier oils, but it is a good addition to blends that will be used in massage mixtures for dry, cracked skin. One part in four of a lighter oil would be a good mix.

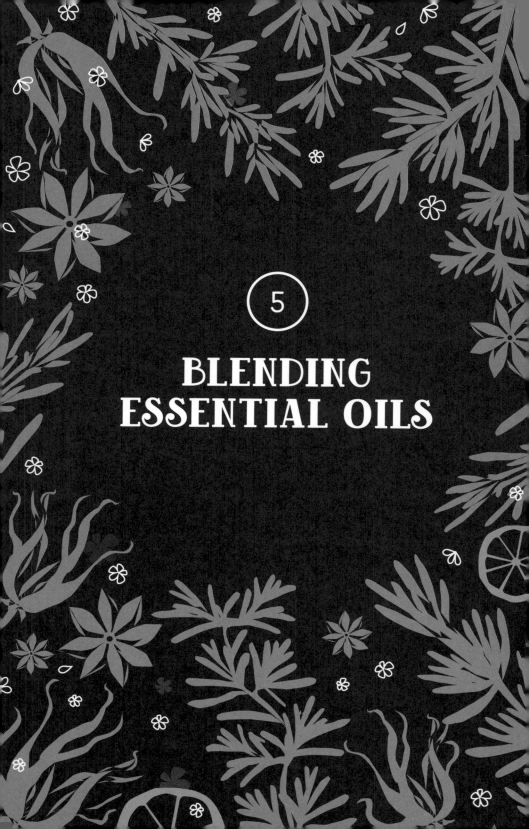

5

BLENDING
ESSENTIAL OILS

> *"Aromatherapy without massage is like an orchestra*
> *without a conductor."*
>
> Robert Tisserand

Essential oils may be used singly or mixed together to make your own personal synergistic blends. These pure essential oils can be blended with any carrier oil (base oil) that you choose to suit your individual taste and according to the purpose that you have in mind. Because essential oils are concentrated and powerful, they must be diluted when used on the skin. Creating different blends is fun, and with experience you will learn which ones suit you best. Why not keep a journal so that you can keep notes of your favorite blends and combinations? The oils I suggest below are my own personal favorites, and they are by no means prescriptive. Your choices may be different! But one suggestion that I would make is to use the oils with the properties that will be useful for the action you require the essential oil to perform.

I have listed some blends to get you off to a start, but try out your own mixtures as well. You can select from a wide range of pure essential oils and natural oil bases that are available in good health stores, and you can enjoy the endless fascination of discovering and creating new blends with these multi-tasking oils.

Stimulating Blend

Use the pure essential oils of rosemary, bergamot, and/or juniper berry in a sweet almond, wheatgerm, and vitamin E base oil. With their strong, refreshing, and purifying aroma, they will stimulate your senses and bring clarity to your mind, especially if you have been experiencing mental fog.

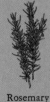
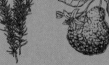

Rosemary   Bergamot   Juniper

Relaxing Blend

Use clary sage and lavender in a grapeseed and vitamin E oil carrier base. With their warming and soothing aromas, this blend is good to use when you are feeling physically and emotionally run-down. This versatile oil blend is good for balancing the mind and body, and if you have trouble sleeping, it can help you get a good night's sleep by encouraging feelings of peacefulness and calm.

Clary Sage   Lavender

Blend to Banish Colds

A good blend to banish colds that are a nuisance and very uncomfortable is the oils of pine, thyme, eucalyptus, or cypress. Choose three of these aromatherapy oils and use them in a body massage, inhalations, or a diffuser.

Thyme   Cypress   Pine   Eucalyptus

Breathe-Easy Blend

Use the head-clearing oils of eucalyptus, peppermint, rosemary, and pine needles in a sweet almond and vitamin E base oil. This blend will help to clear the airways for easy breathing, and it is useful for cold relief. Use during the cold and flu season as a preventative. The antiseptic and invigorating properties of these oils will help you avoid catching the bacterial and viral infections that abound during this season of the year. Inhalation using these oils or using them as a chest rub will help ease breathing when you feel congested.

Peppermint   Rosemary   Pine   Eucalyptus

Sport and Exercise Blend

Three essential oils—eucalyptus, rosemary, and black pepper—blended in a wheatgerm and vitamin E base oil are a good mix to use before taking part in active sports or any exercise, as this strongly fragrant blend will care for the muscles and

Rosemary   Black Pepper   Eucalyptus

tendons, helping to prevent tears. This is a good massage blend if you have overworked and are in need of restoring your vitality.

Enlivening Blend

The pure, refreshing, and stimulating essential oils of pine needles and rosemary, blended in a grapeseed and vitamin E base oil, make an energizing, exhilarating, and activating mixture for the body and mind. It will uplift and restore vigor if you are feeling mentally run-down and will help ease fatigue.

Rosemary   Pine

Improved Well-Being Blend I

The cooling, toning action of geranium and uplifting jasmine, blended with strengthening patchouli, is a mix that will enhance well-being, uplift the mind, and balance the emotions.

Patchouli   Geranium   Jasmine

Improved Well-Being Blend II

The combination of these three fragrant essential oils—geranium, rosewood, and ylang-ylang—blended in a sweet almond and vitamin E base oil will increase feelings of well-being by helping to reduce strain and tension.

 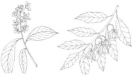

Geranium   Rosewood   Ylang-Ylang

Geranium's sweet, floral fragrance and rosewood's musky and woody aroma, combined with ylang-ylang's euphoric yet relaxing scent, will restore and strengthen the body, helping it to resist infections; steady the emotions; and keep the body systems in balance and harmony.

On-the-Go Blend

If you want to start the morning on a lively note, try using versatile lavender with energizing basil, which helps fight fatigue, along with Roman

Chamomile   Lavender   Basil

chamomile. This is a good first-aid oil mix, blended in a sweet almond and vitamin E base oil. Used first thing in the morning when you shower, this sparkling blend will keep you going from dawn till dusk. This mix is clearing and strengthening to the mind and body, helping the nerves relax and relieving stress.

Sleep-Inducing Blend

For a good night's sleep, try using lavender's balancing energies. This is an excellent oil to help insomniacs relax their frayed nerves and fall asleep easily. Very often

Chamomile   Lavender   Marjoram   Bergamot

this condition is caused by stress and anxiety, and lavender is ideal to use if you suffer from sleep problems. Other calming, soothing oils like chamomile; sweet, warming, sedative marjoram; and relaxing bergamot mixed in a carrier oil of your choice are a good mix to help send you off into a restful slumber. The oils in this blend work with the body to promote calmness, reduce tension and stress, and help relaxation, which is so essential for a restful night.

Try sprinkling the oils onto a handkerchief placed near your pillow, or place the handkerchief on the bedside table for about two to three weeks, replenishing the oils as needed for ongoing benefit.

Room sprays are also a good way to utilize the benefits of these sleep-inducing oils. Used in this way, they may help to reset the body's sleep patterns, which may be out of balance. To make up a room spray, part-fill a clean spray bottle with water, add about ten drops of the essential oils that are proven sleep aids, then shake and spray the room in each of its four corners. Ready-made blends can be purchased in spray bottles and, when empty, you can use them to refill with your own blends. Sweet dreams!

Uplifting Blend

Uplift your spirits with a combination of these wonderful oils: sweet orange, mandarin, petitgrain, or neroli, mixed in a blend of sweet almond and wheatgerm with vitamin E oil. This anti-stress mix will help ease nervous tension, relax the mind, elevate your spirits, and promote positive emotions.

| Mandarin | Petitgrain | Neroli | Orange |

Feminine Hormonal-Balance Blend

Lavender, with its comforting aroma, and soothing Roman chamomile oil, mixed in a blend of sweet almond and natural vitamin E oil, is an ultra-relaxing combination. During times of the month when the body may be out of balance or you're suffering from premenstrual syndrome or menopausal problems, this mix can uplift a low mood, ease depression, and counter that worn-out, run-down feeling.

Chamomile   Lavender

❋ ❋ ❋

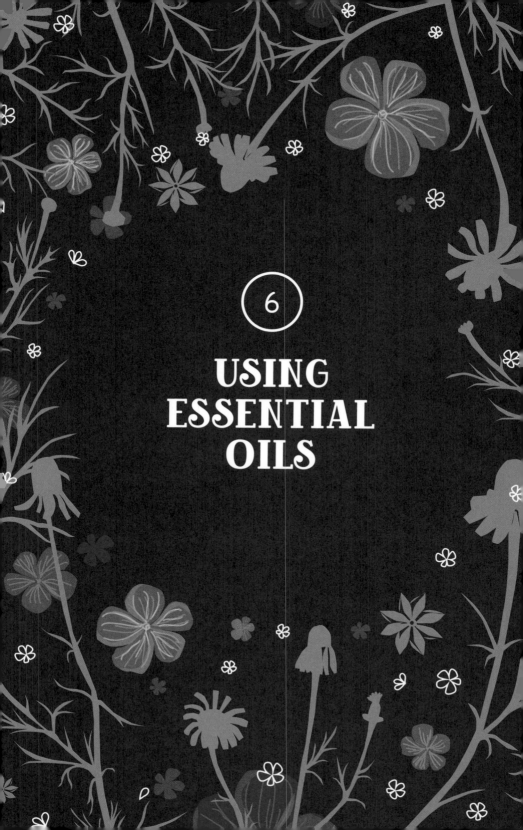

6

USING ESSENTIAL OILS

*"Bread feeds the body, indeed,
but flowers feed the soul."*

The Quran

There are many ways to use essential oils, and you will soon find the methods that suits your lifestyle. With a large variety of oils to choose from, you can treat various conditions or just have a relaxing massage or an aromatic bath, and you can select the appropriate oil for the purpose. Aromatherapy oils work together synergistically. Since these oils contain all the active properties of the plant, they do not have just one use; they have a number of uses over and above their primary function. This is why you will see that one oil—for instance, lavender—will be recommended for a number of conditions and uses. The same applies to all of these therapeutic oils. When you blend the oils with a carrier, you can use up to three oils, depending on which ones are appropriate for your needs. It is best to avoid using more than three oils per blend in any one treatment, as the synergistic effects are less predictable. Add the oils carefully to your blend one at a time.

For example, if you want to have a fragrant bath, the floral oils can be used to soothe you after a tiring day. Choose the three that you wish to use from the floral group: lavender, rose, ylang-ylang, jasmine, or neroli. These lovely flowery oils are not only passive, feminine, cooling, and yielding (yin), but they also give out a heavenly fragrance that is guaranteed to make bath time enjoyable and therapeutic.

The stimulating oils are active, masculine, and resisting (yang), and these are juniper, myrrh, and peppermint. Due to their rousing and stimulating actions, these oils can speed up a sluggish circulation. If you are taking a quick shower in the morning before setting out for the day, you can saturate a washcloth or sponge with a few drops of your chosen invigorating oil—and you will feel ready to meet the day's challenges.

These wonderful oils can be used in inhalations, in diffusers, for massage, and for hand and foot baths. Their use aims to clean and detoxify the body, promote relaxation, and prevent illness by keeping the body's systems in harmony.

Aromatherapists are also aware of the toxicity of certain plants, so care must be taken when using these powerful concentrated substances. Dangerous oils are not generally available for sale to the public.

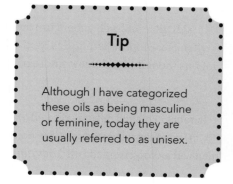

Tip

••••••••••••••

Although I have categorized these oils as being masculine or feminine, today they are usually referred to as unisex.

Bathing for Health, Beauty, and Relaxation

Treatments using aromatherapy baths, water as a healing medium and massage, have been used for thousands of years. Employed for therapeutic purposes as well as for pleasure and enjoyment throughout history, today we can use the same method of application in our own home. Water itself has also been used for "water cures"—and advocated by naturopathic doctors as a "cure" for many ailments. Hydrotherapy is known as "taking the waters," and there is a current revival of interest in this healing system. Expensive health farms provide sauna baths for deep-cleansing—if you are lucky enough to be able to afford a visit. Most people do not have the luxury of staying at an expensive spa, so a bathroom and some tools, essential oils, exfoliators, bristle brushes, and washcloth are all that are needed. This treatment is available to everyone, including those on a tight budget.

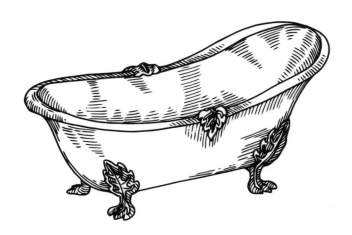

Treatment Bathing and Massage Regimens

You can also "take the waters" in the privacy of your own home spa.

Aromatic Treatment Bath and Massage This is the easiest way to use essential oils at home. What better way to wind down after a stressful and tiring day than to run a luxurious bath filled with aromatic oils, especially if your body aches and your joints creak? There are many oils that can be added to the bath water, helping to cleanse, tone, and beautify your skin, promoting relaxation of your whole body, your mind, and your spirit, while you lie back and soak in the scented water. These treatment baths are designed to help clear up minor ailments and get you back into balance.

Agitate the water before immersing yourself so that the oils can spread evenly. Add up to five drops of your chosen oil to the warm bath water. Make sure you choose oils that do not irritate the skin. If your skin is very dry, dilute the essential oil you wish to use in 2 teaspoons (10ml) of massage base oil before adding to the water for a moisturizing bath.

Stimulating Treatment Bath and Massage Rosemary is a stimulating morning bath additive— invigorating and penetrative. It is good for women's health problems; for example, if you are experiencing menstrual pains, use this oil blended 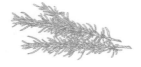 with a carrier of your choice in a morning bath. Follow up with a therapeutic rub, diluting the oil and massaging this mixture over the abdomen, or use it while you are in the bath. This will soothe the pain and will help you get through the day without physical discomfort.

Relaxing Treatment Bath and Massage At the end of a long and stressful day, when you feel tired and washed out, a comforting bath with a few drops of chamomile oil added to the water will help promote relaxation before bedtime. The earthy green fragrance of this delightful oil 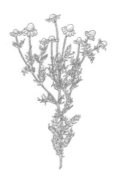 will guarantee a good night's sleep. It is especially useful for anyone who suffers from insomnia, which is often a stress-related condition.

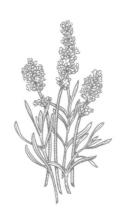

Lavender, with its familiar floral fragrance, is another useful oil to help you drift off to sleep, as is marjoram, with its herbaceous scent. Alternatively, you can use restoring neroli oil and warming, toning, and relaxing clary sage blended into a softening cold-pressed oil of your choice. Good for de-stressing, these two oils blend their energies harmoniously and are good for use at the end of the day to help you unwind. Simply add the blend that you have mixed into the warm running bath water and lie back, relaxing for about fifteen minutes to allow the oils to penetrate your body tissues and to take effect. What could be a more perfect end to a hectic day? Finish off with a body massage using an unperfumed body lotion or cream into which you add a drop or two of lavender or any other floral oil.

Once a week use a body scrub made up of almond oil and sea salt in order to stimulate the circulation, rev up the lymphatic system, and slough off dead skin cells. This will make your skin glow. Follow up with a massage using an unperfumed body lotion to which you have added a few drops of your favorite essential oils. Your skin will thank you for it!

It is best to always blend the oils you have chosen to use with a carrier oil. Make sure you do not use any of the oils that are known irritants, particularly if your skin is sensitive.

Special Care Zones—Feet and Hands

There is nothing more relaxing than a foot soak in a bowl full of warm water and an oil mix of your favorite blend added to it. Tired feet will feel energized after a ten-minute soak in a therapeutic foot bath. The cooling oil of peppermint is particularly therapeutic for hot, aching feet.

Therapeutic Foot Baths If, however, you want to address foot problems, a healing foot bath can help.

Feet take a lot of punishment, and regular foot baths can help to revive your entire system, not just your feet. If you have bunions or inflamed joints, use foot baths regularly to help strengthen and heal the feet; add essential oil of thyme to the blend. When used in massage blends and foot baths, this oil helps to ease stiffness in rheumatic and arthritic joints. Massaging the painful toe-joint called a bunion daily will help alleviate the soreness and swelling.

If you have dry, cracked skin, start off with a preliminary massage using a foot oil blended with a base oil such as almond or avocado. Use a warming, stimulating, and relaxing blend of marjoram, black pepper, and rosemary. After this massage, your feet will already feel much better. Then immerse your feet into a basin of warm water and leave them to soak for about fifteen minutes. Remove your feet and dry them well, then give them another massage using the mixture you made up for the pre-soak blend.

Always combine the oils in an amber-colored glass bottle that is airtight. To emulsify the mixture, shake it vigorously.

Healing Foot Baths If you have a fungal infection such as athlete's foot, you can soak your feet in warm water into which a few drops of the excellent antifungal tea tree oil have been added. This oil is also useful for treating corns and calluses. After a fifteen-minute soak, rinse your feet in a basin of cold water to which you have added some cider vinegar; this has strong cleansing, healing, and germ-fighting properties.

Dry your feet thoroughly, as the fungus that causes athlete's foot thrives in damp areas, and use a new, clean towel every time to reduce the risk of reinfection. Follow up with a therapeutic massage base that blends tea tree with lavender, pine, or rosemary.

Comforting Foot Baths If your feet continually ache and cause pain even though there is no medical problem, use this massage oil blend regularly. After a soak in a foot bath with a few drops of rosemary oil, dry your feet and massage them using a blend of wheatgerm, almond oil, and five drops of rosemary, a penetrating oil that relieves muscle fatigue. Five drops each of black pepper, which relaxes tired muscles, and ginger essential oil are useful as a fortifying tonic for tired, strained muscles. This comforting and soothing regimen of foot baths and massages, carried out as often as time permits, should help alleviate the

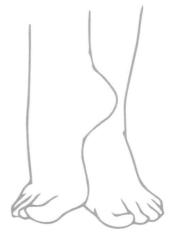

constant aches and pains many people experience due to the amount of weight the feet have to carry.

Therapeutic Hand Baths Hands are as important as feet—and they are always on show. They work very hard and the skin can become dry, sore and cracked. If they are not looked after, they tend to show your age very quickly. Soak your hands for ten minutes in a bowl of hot water to which you have added a few drops of cleansing and refreshing geranium or rose oil, with its delicious fragrance. Dry them thoroughly, then massage them with lashings of a therapeutic hand lotion made up of almond oil and a few drops of sweet, soothing chamomile oil. This will soften and beautify your hands and strengthen your nails.

WHEATGERM-OIL HAND CONDITIONER

- 2 tablespoons (30 ml) of wheatgerm oil or a rich base oil of your choice
- 2 drops of orange essential oil, good for the treatment of eczema and dermatitis
- 1 drop of frankincense oil, one of the most important oils for improving skin tone

Mix the oils together in a small bowl, and then decant them into a dark bottle and store in the fridge.

If your hands are very dry or you have eczema or dermatitis and patches on your hands, this rich mixture will give these areas a chance to heal. Use this homemade hand cream overnight, by spreading it over your hands and then putting on thin cotton gloves. When you wake up in the morning, rinse your hands thoroughly and massage any remaining oil into your hands. Use this therapeutic treatment overnight until the skin heals.

Compresses

A compress is made by placing a cotton cloth into water to which you have added an essential oil, making sure that the essential oil is absorbed by the cloth. Squeeze out the excess water from the cloth, and use the compress to cover the area to be treated. Compresses can be used either hot or cold.

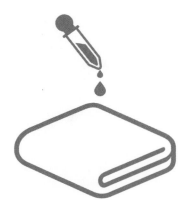

Hot Compress This type of compress draws out poisons from skin infections or eases aches and muscular pains. Hot compresses are good for wherever there is some sort of pain or discomfort.

Most, but not all, conditions that are a type of "ache"—for example, backache, earache, and so on—tend to benefit from hot compresses.

Headaches and migraine do not follow this rule; tension headaches benefit from cold compresses. Use a hot compress *before* an attack of migraine as a preventative, but not during an attack, because people who experience these become hypersensitive during a migraine.

To make a hot compress, fill a bowl with hot water and add two or three drops of the essential oil of your choice. A good pain reliever is lavender, with its mild analgesic properties, or marjoram, with proven analgesic qualities. Place a thin cloth over the surface of the water to soak up the essential oil, wring out the cloth, and apply it to the area that requires treatment. Leave the compress on for about fifteen to twenty minutes, or until it cools down.

Cold Compress This type of compress will ease the pain of sprains, sports injuries, and certain types of headaches as mentioned. Using ice-cold water is best for these types of areas. If the area feels hot and inflamed, a cold compress is ideal. Conditions such as fever and sunburn also benefit from cold compresses.

With experience, you will be able to judge which compress is best to use for the particular injury or condition.

There are also conditions that benefit from alternate hot/cold treatment. Start with a cold compress then alternate with a hot one. Varicose veins benefit from the hot/cold treatment.

Diffusers

Oil Burner/Vaporizer Fill the top of your burner with water and then add an essential oil(s). Light the candle to heat the oil until it evaporates into the atmosphere. The water prevents the oil from overheating, and a few drops of the essential oil of your choice will float on top.

Ultrasonic Diffusers These operate without heat and produce a fine mist with the full quantity of essential oils.

Inhalation This does not require anything elaborate, just a basin with hot water, the essential oils of your choice, and a towel to drape over your head. Inhalation is an instant treatment that can be arranged quickly and easily, for example, if you need to clear airway passages to make breathing easier.

Lightbulb Rings The ceramic rings sit on a lightbulb and heat up. Sprinkle four drops of essential oil of your choice onto the rings to fragrance a room.

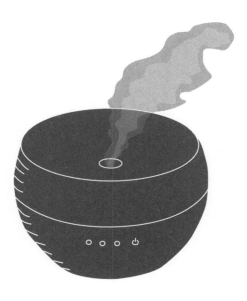

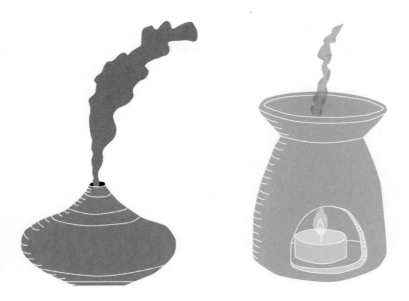

Massage This is an active method used to get an essential oil blend into the skin. Professional aromatherapists use various techniques when massaging a client, depending on the client's problem or condition. If your budget allows it, a visit to a qualified aromatherapist would be a real treat.

Room Sprays These help to purify the air, repel insects, and clear a stuffy nose.

Shower This is a quick and easy way to use essential oils when time is limited.

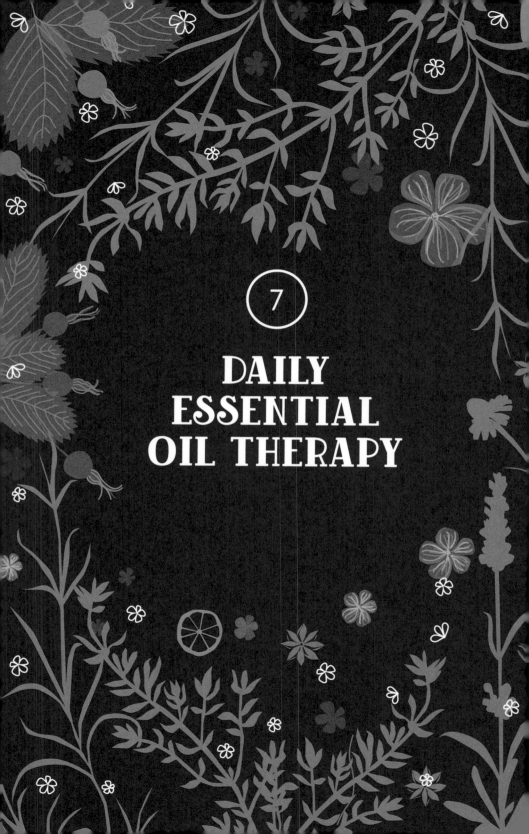

7

DAILY ESSENTIAL OIL THERAPY

"The sense of smell is imagination itself."

Jean-Jacques Rousseau

E xperience the benefits of this healing art as part of your everyday
aromatherapy routine. This regimen will help improve your health,
emotions, and general well-being. Outlined below are daily bathing and shower
rituals for specific moods. Use the oils suggested or the oils of your choice
morning and evening. In this way, you will experience how these valuable oils
can help improve health physically, mentally, and emotionally on a daily basis.
The value of these therapeutic oils is that they can be used in ways that suit
your lifestyle, whatever your age or budget. Keep in mind that most are not
designed to cure any condition, but are used as preventatives, working on the
mind, emotions, and spirit. Enjoy an aroma-soak or shower every day with this
daily routine:

Set the tone for the day with a morning shower that will start you off
feeling positive and ready to face the day. Or at the end of a tiring day, create
a relaxing, calming ambience to help you unwind with an evening bath. Make
it a daily ritual to use aromatherapy oils every day in the shower and bath and
for massage. These oils will keep you in balance and improve your health and
general well-being. If you need to perk up a daily routine, which may have
become a little dull, try an enlivening oil first thing in the morning, when you
take your shower.

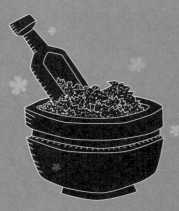

Showers and Baths

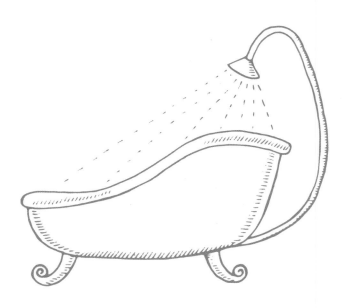

A.M. Shower If you want to be in an uplifted mood all day, have a shower using a plain sea salt scrub with essential oil of orange dropped into the scrub. Orange will help rev up the circulation, is detoxifying, and has a diuretic effect that can reduce water retention and cellulite. Wash the salt scrub off with a body wash of your choice, followed by a chemical-free body lotion. Orange oil's fresh fragrance will revive and awaken you ready for the day to come. You can make up a blend if you choose with other energizing oils. Orange essential oil mixes well with ylang-ylang and rosemary.

P.M. Bath At the end of the day, there's no better way to rebalance yourself than to have a warm soak in the bath using a soothing oil like chamomile—it will help calm any irritability and nervous tension brought on by the stresses of the day. Another soothing oil to use, if you enjoy the sweet, woody fragrance, is cedarwood; this oil will ease tiredness and soothe frazzled

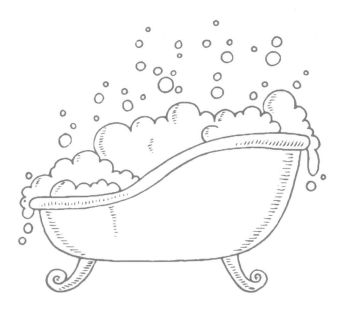

nerves with its clean, sharp aroma. Cedarwood blends well with bergamot's relaxing energies and with sandalwood, a relaxing restorative.

 A.M. Shower If you work in a stressful job and have a hectic lifestyle, lavender essential oil is ideal to use for your morning-shower ritual. Lavender will put you in a calm and harmonizing mood, ready to tackle whatever comes your way. This balancing oil is suitable for all skin types.

To get ready for the busy day ahead, use an exfoliating lotion to which you have added a few drops of lavender, and then wash this off with a lavender-infused body wash. Choose a good-quality body lotion, and you will be ready to face the day feeling pampered. To keep up the good work of your morning ritual, take a handkerchief containing a few drops of lavender oil to work, and sniff this now and again during moments of stress or when the going gets tough, for instance, during a difficult meeting or when working with challenging colleagues.

Lavender oil blends well with pine and citrus oils.

P.M. Bath After a tension-filled day, take a soothing bath into which you have added a few drops of marjoram essential oil. You can use any oil with soothing properties; jasmine or cypress would be ideal. After you finish your bath, follow it up with a massage, which is one of the most self-indulgent ways to enjoy the pleasures of aromatherapy. Make up a massage oil blend with a mixture of your choice. Dilute five drops of one of the suggested oils or one of your favorite oils in 2 teaspoons (10 ml) of a base oil. Then just massage it into your skin at your leisure; this will finish off the day so that you can drift easily into a deep, relaxing sleep.

Always remember that essential oils are very concentrated and they are always diluted in a carrier oil, unless specified as "nonirritant."

 A.M. Shower If you feel that you need to build your confidence for the day ahead and you want to feel alluring inside as well as outside, the use of an oil that has aphrodisiac and invigorating properties will help to strengthen your confidence and self-esteem.

To help you start the day in a confident mood, use a sensual scrub made by adding a few drops of ylang-ylang or rose oil. The heady aromas of these oils promote a sense of well-being, and their use during a morning shower will make you feel marvelous throughout the day.

 P.M. Bath If you are going out on a date in the evening, after a busy day, run a warm bath with an aromatherapy essence that has sensual overtones. Jasmine is a good choice, but any oil whose fragrance you like will suffice. Your aromatherapeutic goal will be to build up your confidence when you go out on the date. After your bath, use a chemical-free body lotion to tone, hydrate, and beautify your body, and use a favorite aromatherapy perfume oil that is redolent of glamour and allure. You can use a nonirritant oil on the skin from the floral range of oils, such as jasmine, rose, or lavender. Don't use too much, and check sensitivity before applying your choice on pulse points.

A.M. Shower If you are one of these people always on the go with no time for yourself, with a busy job, children to look after, and housework to do, you need a revitalizing oil blend that takes you from morning until night.

To kick-start your day, use energizing rosemary, an oil that will awaken and rejuvenate you first thing in the morning. Start with a sea salt scrub to which you have added a couple of drops of rosemary, and wash it off with a chemical-free body wash. Add a body lotion containing a dash of lavender, orange, or pine, any of which blend well with rosemary, but again, go for ones that you enjoy using. This therapeutic morning shower will keep your energy levels up throughout the day.

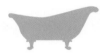 **P.M. Bath** Why not end the day by dropping a few drops of a fragrant aromatherapy oil into warm running water, and then simply lying back and relaxing for ten to fifteen minutes? Incense-like frankincense is a soothing, balancing oil that is emotionally comforting. It blends well with the spice oil, myrrh, and warm, woody sandalwood, as well as with sensuous patchouli. Lie back in the fragrant waters, enjoying the sybaritic pleasure of some "me-time"—you deserve it!

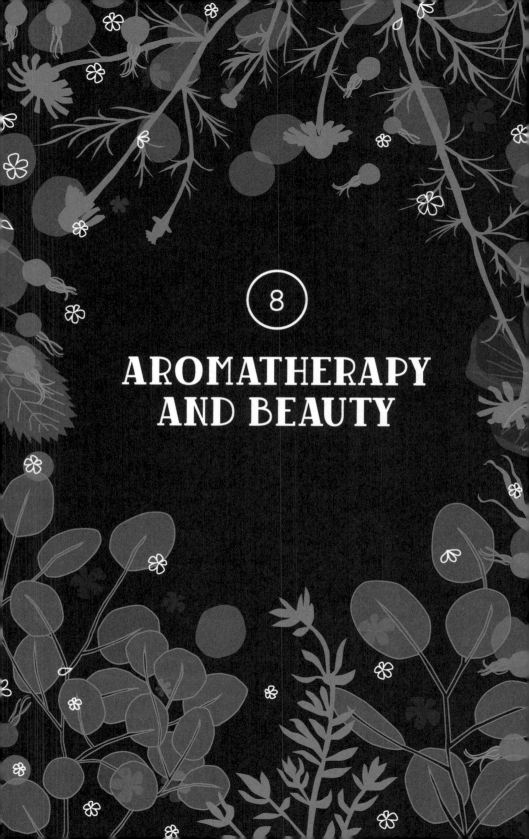

8

AROMATHERAPY AND BEAUTY

"Scents are surer than sights and sounds to make your heart strings crack."

Rudyard Kipling

Skin Care

The essential oils extracted from many marvelous plants are particularly valuable for use in skin care. They can be used for all kinds of skin conditions and problems. Choose certified organic or natural oils, as these do not contain any chemicals. It is the pure essential oils that become a concentrated essence after distillation that work best in holistic beauty care.

Nature's beauty essences used for skin maintenance act quickly and effectively to rebalance the epidermis, which is the outer layer of the skin. If the skin is too oily or too dry, it can be brought back into balance. The texture of beauty oils is much finer and more easily absorbed than shop-bought creams and lotions. Only a tiny quantity is required, due to their incredibly concentrated form, which makes them so effective and easy to use.

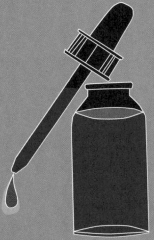

Unscented lotions or creams can be mixed with essential oils. Two or three drops in an unperfumed cream or lotion is all you need. Using these oils regularly will improve any skin condition and give the skin a healthy, radiant glow.

There are many different essential oils that you can use in your beauty regimen. Decide into what category your skin falls, and then choose the right oil for your skin type.

Skin Types

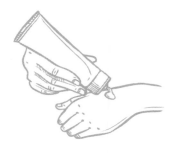

Dry Skin Dry skin can tend to look tired and dull. It may have fine lines and appear dehydrated. This type of skin needs repair using only the purest plant oils. A couple of drops of a pure essential oil in a rosehip oil carrier is rich in antioxidants, or drop the pure plant oil of your choice in a plain cream and use it to moisturize your face and neck. Alternatively, you can massage rosehip oil directly into your face and neck before you apply your chosen cream or lotion. This will hydrate and nourish, while also protecting your skin from free-radical damage.

Another oil that is very good as a carrier for dry skin is the oil from the avocado. This is a rich and unrefined oil, high in the powerful antioxidant vitamin E. Too rich to use on its own, avocado oil is very good as a carrier when mixed with another base. Two or three drops of frankincense, known for its rejuvenating qualities, can be added. This pure essential oil has long been used in facial blends to help prevent fine lines and wrinkles, to which dry skin is prone. This blend, with its rich vitamin content, will nourish dry, devitalized skin.

Normal Skin Not many women are lucky enough to have a normal skin that is in perfect balance, with fine pores and a smooth and even texture. Although this skin type is clear and fine grained, it still needs to be looked after, as it can easily lose its suppleness and flawless appearance. Good oils to use to keep normal skin balanced would be a blend of three drops each of rose, frankincense, and neroli mixed in 2 teaspoons (10 ml) of a light oil, such as apricot-kernel, and two teaspoons of jojoba. These two carriers work well together and easily penetrate the skin.

Oily and Combination Skin Oily skin is usually linked to hormonal changes during puberty or menopausal changes later in life. Men can also experience oily skin during puberty. Combination skin is a common type, and it is easily recognizable: usually the cheeks are prone to dryness and the T-zone is shiny and oily. This type of skin is thought to be due to an acid condition.

A good base oil to use for greasy skin is grapeseed. It is light and odorless and has a nongreasy texture. Another carrier for treating greasy skin is jojoba, as it is a balancing oil.

Combination skin can benefit from using a blend of 4 teaspoons (20 ml) of a balancing jojoba base with the addition of two balancers—lavender (three drops) and geranium (three drops)—with the addition of detoxifying sweet orange oil (three drops).

If there is any sign of acne, a blemished-skin blend is useful, made up of juniper oil for its astringent and detoxifying properties, mixed with lavender, chamomile, or lemon with its purifying qualities and lymphatic cleansing ability. Note that lemon can be an irritant for some people and may increase sensitivity to sunlight. Do not use a strong concentration.

Mature Skin For the purpose of skin rejuvenation, essential oils are pretty remarkable. They contain potent rejuvenating substances extracted from aromatic plants. To avoid any irritation, these oils must always be diluted in a suitable carrier oil before being applied to the skin.

Mature skin needs an anti-ageing regimen in order to prevent lines and wrinkles and reduce the appearance of any that have already appeared. Many essential oils help regenerate skin cells and stimulate cellular activity. They can tone the skin, helping to reduce fine lines and wrinkles. Another problem with ageing skin is the appearance of discoloration and age spots; this is often caused by sun damage due to sunbathing without applying sunblock.

NOURISHING CARRIER FOR AGEING AND MATURING SKIN

Macadamia oil has a rich fatty acid composition, so it is ideal for use when diluting the aromatherapy essences that will be used in a base oil due to its soft, silky texture and its quick absorption into the skin. Used regularly, this blend will make ageing skin respond with renewed life.

All skin will benefit from regular mini-facials and steaming, because the hot vapor helps to open pores and remove impurities. Regular gentle exfoliation is also beneficial, so that the upper cellular debris on the epidermis can be removed. This allows the skin to appear clearer, with a clean base, which will make it more receptive to any moisturizing or oil treatments that will be applied.

Choose a good carrier like argan oil, which is high in omega fatty acids, and mix it with another rich carrier oil. Helpful aromatherapy oils to add for this type of skin are frankincense, a balsamic firming rejuvenator known for its regenerating qualities; lavender, which is a cell regenerator; and neroli, a nourishing, replenishing oil that is ideal for mature complexions. Patchouli is a tissue-generating oil useful for skin that has begun to wrinkle. Growing older is inevitable, but age does not matter as long as you don't look it! Youthful maturity is the aim, and with the regular use of nature's finest oils, you can retain the beauty of your skin for years to come.

Skin Elixirs and Serums

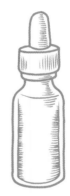

Plant serums are used in holistic skin care as therapeutic agents and they work well, due to their similarity to the skin's epidermis. Making a plant serum at home is not difficult. You can custom-blend these skin conditioners yourself, using good-quality ingredients. Only use plant oils as a carrier or base oil; they are used to dilute the essential oils and to support their use in a therapeutic blend. Once the serum or elixir is mixed, put it in dark bottles and store them away from light. Shake well before use.

All of these serums and elixirs can be used in conjunction with a facial massage.

Dry and Sensitive Nourishing Skin Elixir

- 2 tablespoons (30 ml) apricot-kernel oil – suitable for mature, dry, and sensitive or inflamed skin
- 3 drops of lavender essential oil – calms and balances skin, allowing it to regenerate naturally
- 3 drops of geranium oil – regenerates new skin cells, boosts circulation, and has scar-reducing properties
- 2 drops of rose oil – a great skin healer, full of antioxidants

This nourishing elixir, used before your moisturizer during the day or before your night cream, will help to calm and moisturize your skin, improve tone and texture, and make dry and sensitive skin feel more comfortable.

Rejuvenating Facial Serum
- 2 teaspoons (10 ml) jojoba or macadamia oil, both suitable for facial blends
- 4 drops of frankincense oil, known for its rejuvenating properties
- 2 drops of lavender oil, suitable for most skin types
- 2 drops of geranium oil, a good skin balancer

This nutritious and skin-supporting serum can be used on all skin types before moisturizer is applied and before night cream.

Caution With sensitive skin, always do a patch test first.

Anti-Ageing Serum
- 1 teaspoon (5ml) macadamia oil, quickly absorbed by the skin; its honeyed texture benefits most skin types, particularly mature complexions.
- 1 teaspoon (5ml) rosehip oil, a superb rejuvenating oil with a fine texture.
- 4 drops frankincense oil, important for treating ageing skin and wrinkles and for preventing skin ageing if used early enough.

Any anti-ageing skin care serum can be used from the early thirties on. The skin starts to age on a cellular level quite early in life, and aromatherapy oils in various blends are very good at preventing signs of ageing, dark spots, and so on.

Skin Protective Elixir
- 1 teaspoon (5ml) avocado oil mixed with sweet almond oil – a regenerating and stimulating blend that will revitalize dull skin due to its high concentration of vitamins and essential fatty acids.
- 4 drops lavender
- 3 drops geranium

This calming elixir is suitable for dry, sensitive, irritated skin and can be used before a moisturizer and before a night cream.

❋ ❋ ❋

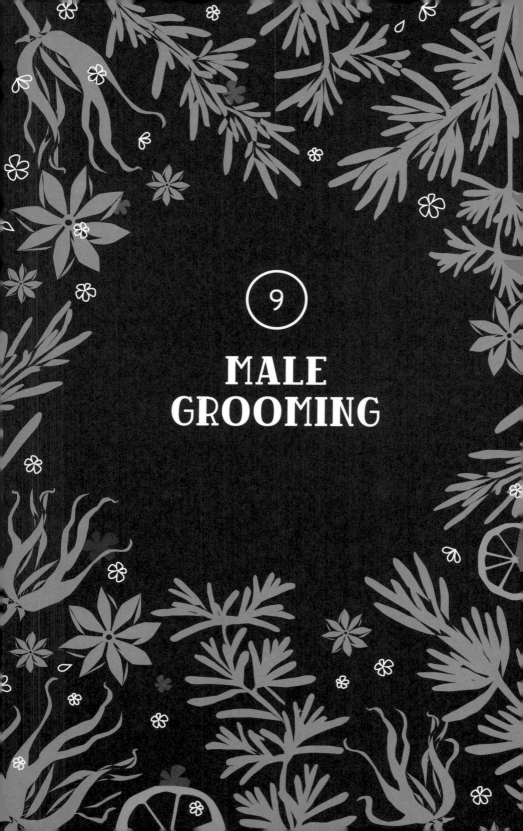

9

MALE
GROOMING

"Aromatherapy is extremely useful. If you want to sleep at night and you have an aroma that calms your mind, it will help you sleep."

Deepak Chopra

Aromatherapy is suitable for men as well as women. At last men can look after their appearance and grooming without this being seen as only for women. Men matter!

Men's interest in the use of natural products to improve their health and looks has finally arrived. They are turning away from chemically laden personal care formulations made in a laboratory and are choosing instead all-natural skin and bath products made with nature's extracts. Aromatherapy offers a wide range of therapeutic oils to help improve the health and appearance of men's facial and body skin.

For men who shave daily, the use of grooming products made up of natural oils can be invaluable in helping to improve skin health along with general health. With frequent use of these essences, men will recognize the real benefits of aromatherapy oils. By using them regularly, they will see improvements in their skin, body, and hair, as well as in their general well-being.

Pre-Shave Oils

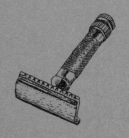

Using pre-shave aromatherapy oils each morning will turn a shave into a treatment instead of a form of medieval torture! Daily shaving can cause skin irritation and razor burn or simply leave the skin feeling itchy, uncomfortable, and dry. Mixing a soothing mixture of lavender oil, with its mild analgesic properties, and comforting chamomile in a nourishing vegetable oil like apricot-kernel, will provide relief if the skin has become sore and red after daily shaving. If you use a razor, always make sure that it is sharp, and shave only in the direction of your hair growth. If your skin is on the oily side, oil of lemon with its antibacterial and astringent qualities in a light carrier oil will cleanse the skin and reduce the production of sebum (an oily product of the sebaceous glands).

If there are any spots or blemishes, a dab of neat tea tree oil with its disinfectant properties will help to clear these up.

Steam Cleanse If you suffer from acne, blemishes, or congested skin, first look to your diet. Often hormone fluctuations or a poor state of health may be the reason, but it can be hard to find the reason the skin overreacts this way. Using facial steam cleansing once or twice a week to clear blocked pores and purify the skin will help. Drop a couple of cleansing essential oils, such as tea tree or lemon, into the hot water in a facial sauna, or use a bowl of hot water with a towel draped over your head for about two or three minutes. Gentle, antiseptic grapefruit oil in a blend can be applied after the facial steam treatment to tone and tighten the skin, or to clear oily skin.

Regular use of a lavender and chamomile mixture will help with any ingrown hairs that may occur when the hair follicle is damaged by poor grooming practices. There will be an improvement in skin texture and tone. Treating the skin with a mild exfoliating cream once a week will loosen ingrown hairs and slough off any buildup of cellular debris. The skin should be glowing after weekly exfoliating treatments.

If you wish to add other essential oils to your daily shaving ritual, lemon balm—also known as melissa—is useful if facial skin is inflamed. This oil is excellent for skin care.

Blotchiness and Flaky Skin If blotchy red patches appear on facial skin due to the use of an old, dull razor blade, or the skin has become flaky and dry, use a mixture of anti-inflammatory chamomile and antiseptic bergamot; if you wish, add calming lavender to the mix in a nourishing carrier like almond oil. This blend is good for all skin types, and it is especially gentle on sensitive skin. With regular use, the skin will return to its normal state of balance.

Natural Aftershave Balm

Make up an aftershave balm using a plain, unperfumed lotion with the addition of a few drops of essential oils of your choice. The masculine aromas of citrusy bergamot, pine-fresh juniper berry, and sweet, exotic, lingering sandalwood are good to use. This healing balm, with its natural restoring and conditioning properties, will leave the skin moisturized and feeling comfortable, especially if facial skin has become sore and dry from daily shaving. An added bonus will be the fresh, masculine aroma of this woody, peppery aftershave balm, blended with a hint of fresh-smelling citrus. These days, scent is considered unisex, so there are fragrances that appeal to both men and women.

You may like to try adding other oils with a masculine fragrance to your natural aftershave balm. For instance, try black pepper, bay, vetiver, frankincense, and cedarwood. Have fun experimenting with different mixes until you find the one you like best! These aromas are wonderfully uplifting and mood enhancing.

Beard Oils

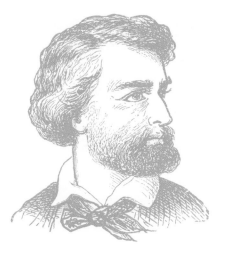

If you have a beard, there are a number of beard oils made up of nourishing base oils and essential oils with fragrances that appeal to men. A number of carriers can be used, according to your skin type:

- Argan oil is valued for its nutritive properties.
- Avocado is a rich base oil that works well blended with other base oils.
- Sweet almond helps to soothe itching and sore skin.
- Jojoba oil soothes skin and helps to unclog hair follicles.

Choose an essential oil and blend it with one more base. Essential oils of earthy cedarwood and sweet, woody sandalwood go well together, or, if you prefer, add the fresh smell of pine. Lavender and rosemary are good partners and blend well. It is up to you; the main aspect of beard maintenance is to stop the beard looking unkempt.

Mix the oils in a small, dark bottle that has a cap or eyedropper. Shake the bottle well. To apply, put a few drops into your hands, rub them together, and then rub the mixture through the beard and onto the cheeks.

After your morning shower, sprinkle a few drops of the beard oil in your hands, rub together and apply. Just before going to bed at night, follow the same ritual, and your beard will benefit from the same conditioning benefits overnight that it did during the day.

Bath

Luxuriate in a warm bath after a tiring day at work, after a session at the gym, or after a sports day. Drop an essential oil mixed with a base oil into the bath water, then lie back and enjoy the soak. A good blend would be black pepper for its energizing properties (possible irritant; do not use in concentrations above 0.5 percent, and do a patch test). Use cedarwood with its soothing and toning qualities to help relieve aches and pains, or frankincense for its rejuvenating and energizing benefits. The green fragrance of cypress is also considered a "masculine" smell.

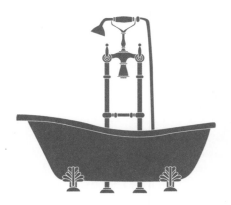

Shower

In the morning a quick invigorating shower with a few essential oils of your choice sprinkled on a sponge or washcloth will help to stimulate and revitalize you before you head out for the day. Use a light body lotion after every shower or bath to condition the skin and supplement your skin's natural protection. You will notice a definite improvement with regular use.

Hair Care

Before you shampoo your hair, prepare the massage oil. Blend a mixture of sweet almond oil, good for all skin types and gentle on problem and sensitive skins, with jojoba oil suitable for hair preparations. Add a few drops of stimulating rosemary oil. Massage your head and scalp, using both hands and starting at the back of the head, and work around the sides and over the top. This will encourage blood circulation, treat dandruff, and also stimulate good hair development. Done regularly, this may help to prevent thinning, hair loss, and baldness, which are common problems for men that can result in a lack of confidence. Shampoo the hair and then rinse thoroughly. Massage the hair to remove the last bits of shampoo, and rinse twice more.

Juniper oil has antiseptic anti-dandruff and sebum-regulating properties. Massaged into the scalp with a light base, it will encourage healthy hair.

Essential oils are absorbed into the scalp. Add cedarwood essence to the blend, as this oil blends well with rosemary, and it will help to improve oily skin and itchy scalp.

Regular use of these natural plant essences, combined with natural plant bases, will help keep hair and scalp healthy and smelling fresh and clean.

Sports and Exercise

After exercising or a sports day, massage is the traditional solution to muscular aches and pains. If you belong to a sports club, a massage by a professional masseuse would be a wonderful treat. If not, try a self-treatment with an invigorating muscle rub made up of a base oil and the essential oils of thyme, pine, and cedarwood. This moisturizing, warming, invigorating, and comforting balm will not only relax and soothe muscles, it will also improve well-being.

Sleep

If you have trouble sleeping at night, with your mind not turning off, worrying about work or any other problems, a couple of drops of calming lavender on your pillow will send you off into a soothing slumber ready to wake refreshed the next day.

❈ ❈ ❈

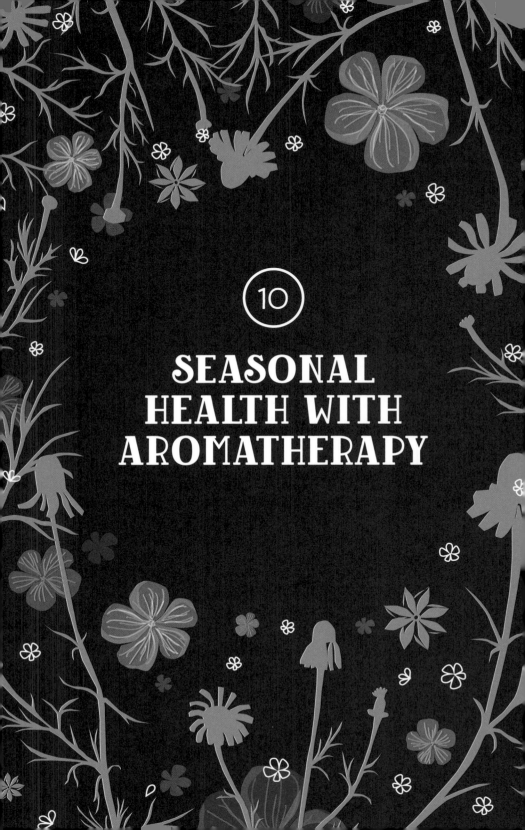

10

SEASONAL
HEALTH WITH
AROMATHERAPY

> *"Nature bestows her own, richest gifts and with lavish*
> *hands, she works in shifts."*
>
> Gertrude Tooley Buckingham

Each season of the year relates to our health and well-being. Taking steps before the next season or during it will help us to live in balance with nature's forces. Aromatherapy is one of the simplest and gentlest complementary therapies that can be used at home, in any season, to keep well. Poet Gertrude Tooley Buckingham was right when she said that nature works in shifts!

Many health conditions are impacted by the seasons, and there is a seasonal variance in health and illness. With every changing season comes a shift of energy, and health-supporting essential oils can be used therapeutically and also as a preventative throughout the year. Energy constantly changes and flows, and the energies of the body also change with each passing season. So you should change your health regimen with the yearly energy flow—this way, the energy movements of the body can tune in harmoniously with nature's yearly cycles. Just like the changing yearly energies, the body has its own cycles and rhythms. Following different health regimens at different times of the year will help attune our energies harmoniously with nature's creative forces and changing weather patterns.

Here are some of my favorite oils for each season of the year. You can use these as a starting point for your own experiments with aromatherapy. Always buy good-quality oils, because cheaper oils are often adulterated and will not work therapeutically. Many oils complement each other and can be mixed together to make creative blends.

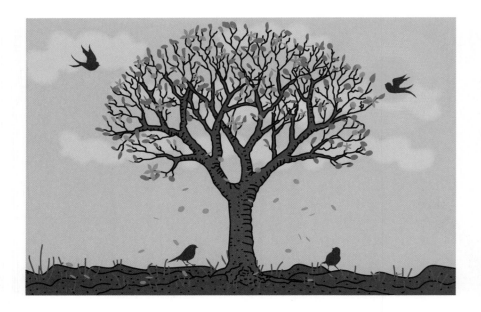

Spring

At this time of the year, the dormant energies of winter gradually awaken into spring. The thrusting vibrant energies of springtime, a time of new beginnings, bring forth new life. It is a time of renewal, when all around young shoots and buds appear on plants and trees. Unfortunately, this is also the pollen season, and many people suffer from allergies and hay fever at this time. These are uncomfortable and debilitating conditions that can last for weeks, with sore, itchy eyes and endless sneezing. Prevention is the best cure, and the use of essential oils before spring arrives is the best method of helping to avert these problems.

Oils to use before spring begins are chamomile, lemon balm, lavender, or pine in a soothing bath or in inhalations, as this can help with mucus and catarrh. If used regularly, this preventative measure may ease the misery of these conditions, as long as it is started early enough. If this does not help, then during the season, a blend of cleansing eucalyptus and calming lavender may prove helpful in a steam inhalation or as a massage blend, or you could sprinkle a few drops onto a handkerchief to be inhaled during the day. These conditions can also be helped with good nutrition and dietary changes.

It makes sense to boost your immune system before the onset of the pollen season. Preparing the body with a course of bee pollen prior to the hay-fever season is sensible. Bee pollen is nature's own balancing substance, and it can be used as a de-sensitizing medium before the season begins, as it has been known to lessen symptoms. Hay-fever sufferers are allergic to inhaled pollens, but surprisingly, bee pollen, which is rich in vitamins, minerals, and amino acids, appears to be successful in ameliorating attacks during the pollen season. By taking bee pollen for a month or two prior to the hay-fever season, the body apparently becomes de-sensitized to grass pollens and clouds of flower pollens. Unless you are allergic to bee products, it might be worth a try.

Detoxing

Cleansing diets to rid the body of stored wastes can be used once or twice a year, and this season of new beginnings is the ideal time to start. After the comfort foods of winter, you should begin a healthful regimen to support the cleansing processes of the body of accumulated toxins. This is a time to get yourself in gear after the passive energies of winter when the body has usually been wrapped up in heavy clothing and the skin may look dull. This is the time to start a lighter, healthier diet full of fresh, wholesome foods that will help cleanse the body internally. You can also use various detoxing oils that help eliminate excess weight gain and improve skin tone, getting you ready to expose more skin as the weather warms up. You will enjoy wearing lighter clothes with confidence after a couple of weeks of detoxing with diet and aromatherapy.

Used in therapeutic baths or massage blends, healing oils can help to free the body of impurities and improve health. After a detox, you will feel more energetic, your skin will look clearer and more youthful, and you will feel better. A detox may also encourage natural weight loss if weight was gained during the winter. You will enjoy increased vitality and increased seasonal well-being.

To maximize the effects of the bath, dry-brush your skin with a natural-fiber brush before bathing to open up pores and remove dead skin cells. Spend a few minutes doing this before you enter the bath. Always work toward the heart area when brushing the skin. Now you will be ready to enjoy a good soak in the fragrant waters of the bath you have prepared. Use about four drops of essential oil in a bath filled halfway, or six to eight in a full bath.

When you are submerged in the luxurious waters, massage your skin with gentle, circular motions to bring blood to the surface. In addition to improving circulation, a massage will tone muscles and energize the body. You can, if you wish, use a loofah or vegetable sponge; this is the dry, fibrous part of a gourd.

It is a very effective way to cleanse the whole body, and, once wet, the loofah swells up and can thoroughly cleanse areas that are prone to spots, such as the chest and back.

Give Yourself a Spring Clean

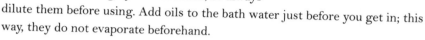

Detox baths accelerate toxic elimination, removing wastes and cellular debris. Bathing can encourage your body to sweat the toxins out. Essential oils are highly concentrated, so always dilute them before using. Add oils to the bath water just before you get in; this way, they do not evaporate beforehand.

Detox Bath Use a jar of plain bath salts or fine sea salts and add a few drops of detoxifying, regenerating lemon oil, along with a couple of drops of fresh, green rosemary oil. Grapefruit oil can be substituted for any one of these oils; it is diuretic and decreases unwanted mucus during detoxification. This oil may be an irritant for some, so do a patch test before use.

Detox Bath Use a jar of plain bath salts or fine sea salts and add a few drops of lemongrass, an oil that is good for drainage of body fluids, and calming lavender oil. Do not bathe for longer than twenty minutes, as bathing for longer than this will dry out the skin. Avoid high concentrations of this oil.

Detox Bath Juniper oil helps detox the body by ridding it of toxic wastes, improving elimination, and supporting liver function. Add it to a cup of fine sea salts, as these salts encourage sweating, which is another way the body eliminates toxins. Juniper is nonirritating in dilution.

During the detox regimen, add two drops of juniper on the pulse points of the wrists each day and inhale its stimulating aroma. This oil helps tone up the glandular system, particularly the pancreas and adrenals.

Caution Do not use juniper oil if you have a kidney disorder. You can try grapefruit oil, as it supports liver and lymphatic cleansing, but only use a low concentration.

Essential oils for spring are uplifting, energizing, and stimulating. Lemon and lemongrass, with their citrusy aroma; marjoram, with its herbaceous scent; and melissa, known as lemon balm, with its lemony fragrance—all have a spring-like feel about them.

A refreshing body massage during spring is perfect for anyone feeling tired and in need of revitalization. A special blend of mandarin, lemon, orange, or ylang-ylang in a softening carrier oil base that is massaged all over the body is a therapeutic experience, and you can concentrate on tired areas that need extra help. Absorption of the oils into the skin will enhance their therapeutic effect. You do not have to use all four oils in one blend; it is best to use no more than three oils, because the synergistic blend of too many oils can be unpredictable. Experiment with the blends, using oils with cleansing properties.

Summer

Summer is nature's season of maturity—a time of the year when hot "yang" energies can be overwhelming, and we take a break from work with holidays and relaxation. It is a time when the driving energies of spring begin to mellow, but seasonal allergies can still persist during summer. Follow the detox regimen suggested for spring.

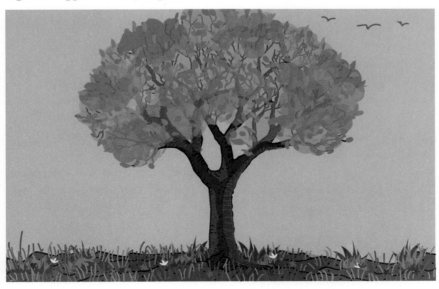

Summertime is an uplifting season, when energies are bubbly and vivacious and we feel more alive. The hot sun makes people feel better and uplifted. A lot of recreational activities take place, people spend time basking in sunshine, and the outdoor life sustains us. During this time of year, vitamin D is created as the body synthesizes this vitamin from the ultraviolet rays that are absorbed into the skin. This is the season when vitamin D status is at its highest, but care must be taken to avoid staying in the sun without protection. This is also a time when plenty of salads and fruits are enjoyed, which makes weight loss easier.

Summer requires aromatherapy oils to help the body cool off. Geranium oil with its fresh, cooling properties, or cooling, toning, and balancing palmarosa, can be used when taking a shower. Sprinkle a couple of drops of rose-scented geranium or sweet, musky palmarosa onto a washcloth or a sponge and take a refreshing shower during the heat of this season. Used in a a cream, this is a first-rate massage medium for those who prefer an alternative to massage oils during summer. The benefits will be felt both physically and mentally.

This is the time of year when the solar energy beaming down on us makes us all feel better. Sunny days and balmy nights are a time when we feel carefree, a time when we are more active and likely to be living the outdoor life.

Autumn

At this the time of the year, summer's strong energies are beginning to wane and a big shift in energy takes place. It is time to begin to get back to work after the lazy days of summer. Adapt your diet to suit this season of the harvest, and plan for the coming winter with a wholesome diet and strengthening oils to help build and prepare the body for the colder months to come. If you improved your vitamin D status during the summer months, this will help protect you during the coming months of colder weather. It is around this time that colds and coughs and other health conditions brought on by damp weather begin to appear. If you have kept in tune with the ebbs and flows of the changing year's cycles, your immune system will have been strengthened. You will have prepared yourself for the shorter days of autumn with your cleansing regimens and detoxification, so you should get fewer colds and bouts of the flu, having primed up your immune system.

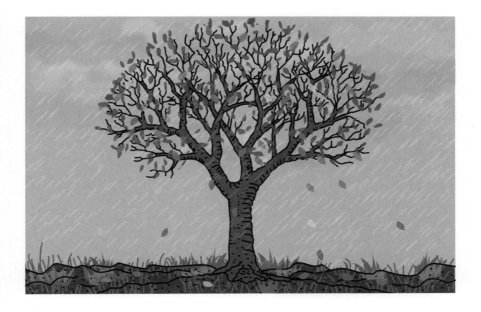

Autumn oils that are strengthening can be used in baths, for massage or diffusion, or blended in base oil.

Patchouli is a strengthening and stimulating oil with an exotic floral aroma. Use patchouli therapeutically during this season to help build up strength before the coming winter, so that you can fight off viruses and bacterial infections. If you do catch a cold or come down with the flu, a few drops of camphorated eucalyptus in a steam inhalation and as a chest and throat rub will help shorten the illness's duration.

Keeping to a healthy whole-food diet with plenty of seasonal fruits and vegetables rich in vitamin C and beta carotene will build up your immune system, which is so important at this time of the year. If you skip a few days without eating nutritious food, take a good-quality vitamin and mineral supplement made from a whole-food base to provide all the nutrients the body needs. You must keep your immune system fortified. This regimen will help build you up to face the winter's coming cold temperatures and dark days.

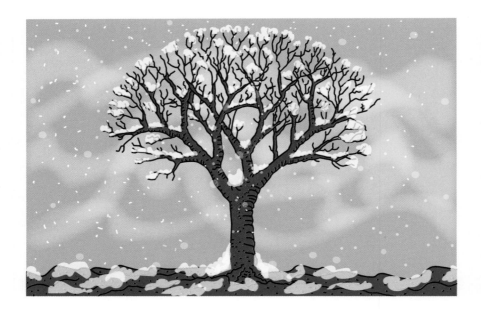

Winter

During the winter months, our energies begin to wind down. This is a time of year when colds, flu, and cold "yin" illnesses are prevalent. Nearly everyone succumbs, but with seasonal preparation you should be able to avoid catching anything serious. Warming "yang" essential oils are ideal to be used throughout the winter.

Winter warming oils have a lovely rich, spicy fragrance that helps to get you into the spirit of the winter season. Regular use of warming oils during the winter months will enhance your well-being, allowing you to enjoy this time of the year relatively problem free. Ginger is effective for winter chills and it is a healing balm for sore, aching muscles, bringing warmth when applied to a painful area. During this time of year when energies are low, ginger added to a diffuser will create a flow of spicy fragrance throughout the air. Ginger helps to move cold, "stagnant" energies, thus improving circulation. Do not use ginger on the skin undiluted or in baths as it can be an irritant.

Another warming oil is black pepper. Its intense properties and pungent smell, blended with a base oil to create a muscle rub, will get the circulation moving and ease stiff joints, general aches and pains, and colds. Alternatively, add this essential oil to a warm aromatherapy bath (remembering the cautions about each essential oil) during winter. During a bath, the therapeutic actions of these precious oils are two-fold: they are absorbed through the skin and can enter the circulatory system, which can become sluggish during winter. The added bonus is that their aromas are inhaled, increasing feelings of warmth and well-being.

In the cold winter months, when we are covered up with heavy clothes, the skin tends to become dry and the circulation sluggish. Start off with a skin-brushing session before taking a shower, and then use appropriate stimulating aromatherapy oils on a sponge or washcloth. This will stimulate circulation and improve lymphatic drainage, which in turn will improve skin texture. This method exfoliates dead top skin layers, helps regenerate cells, and allows body lotions and creams to be absorbed more easily.

For toning the skin, use refreshing cypress. For a stimulating shower, use cleansing and energizing pine or toning essence of rosemary. During this time of the year, lymphatic congestion can become a problem, so geranium, with its soothing and balancing qualities, used regularly with a friction mitt, will help improve lymphatic drainage. Do not rub too hard if skin is sensitive. If carried out regularly, this regimen will also help get the circulation going. If you can stand it, an invigorating cold shower afterward will help stimulate the lymphatic system, getting it moving and boosting circulation and cleansing the system of toxic wastes as well. If you are using pine oil, avoid high concentrations, as sensitization is possible.

Do not use the above oils without first blending them in a carrier base, and be careful not to use too much, as they are very concentrated and can irritate sensitive skin.

❋ ❋ ❋

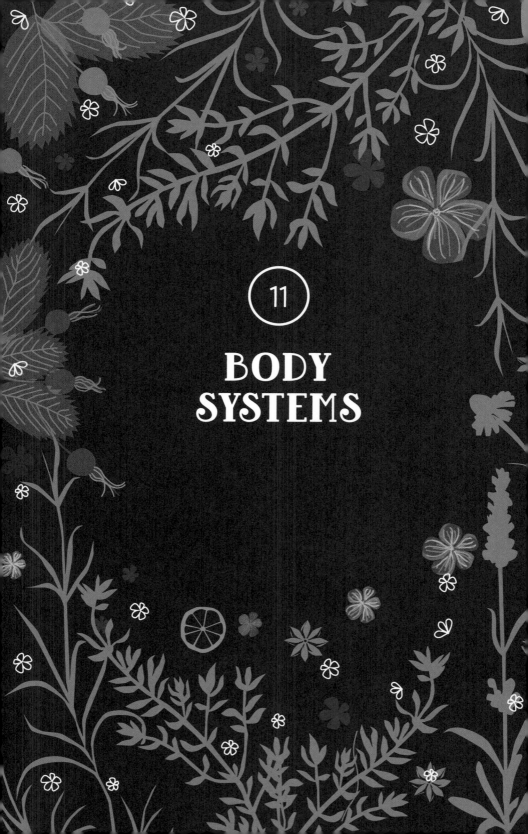

11

BODY SYSTEMS

"One touch of Nature makes the whole world kin."

William Shakespeare

Aromatherapists are trained to view the mind, body, and spirit as a whole, and they treat their clients in a holistic way. When one part of the body is out of balance, it is a reflection of disharmony within the whole system. This is in tune with the Hippocratic philosophy of a holistic approach to health that brings about balance between mind, body, and spirit. Using the appropriate oils with massage techniques and other treatments, an aromatherapist can help to unify their client's mind, body, and spirit.

People consult aromatherapists for any number of health reasons, including prevention, in order to keep the body and mind in good health and balance. They also consult them for a wide range of beauty treatments. Nothing is more relaxing than a soothing aromatic massage by a skilled therapist, or a facial using aromatic beauty oils.

Specific essential oils have an affinity with certain organs and body systems, and when using essential oils at home for minor ailments, there are several ways to enjoy their benefits. They can be used for massage, which is the most popular method, as it enables absorption of the oils into the skin. Dilute your choice of essential oils in a base oil at the recommended proportion, which is usually about five drops to every 2 teaspoons (10 ml) of base oil. You can use these oils in the bath or vaporization to create different moods in the home. These are just some of the ways in which these versatile aromatherapy oils can be used to give pleasure and to enhance health and well-being.

This chapter deals with various types of mild health complaints and ways in which aromatherapy can help to treat them. For each problem, recommendations are made for essential oils, carrier bases and blends, and the various methods of application.

The Circulatory System

This system of the body consists mainly of the heart and a series of tubes that carry substances to and from different areas of the body. Every cell in the body must receive nourishment provided by the bloodstream. This system removes wastes via the kidneys, intestines, skin, and lungs. Aromatherapy places great emphasis on taking preventative measures, its philosophy being an ounce of prevention is worth a pound of cure, and the circulatory system needs attention in order to prevent heart disease and related problems.

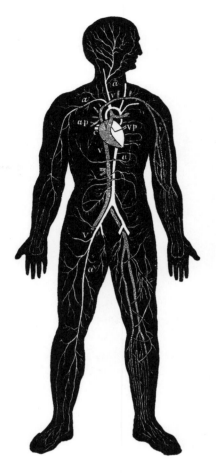

High Blood Pressure

Many people suffer from this condition, particularly in the West. Dietary factors play a large part in elevating blood pressure, as do stress, alcohol, too much salt, lack of exercise, and smoking. Some serious disorders that require medical attention are diseases of the kidneys and complications during pregnancy. These conditions can elevate blood pressure, and they are serious problems that must be dealt with by a medical doctor.

If blood pressure has become elevated due to stress or stress-related conditions such as nervous tension or anxiety, the following blends can help alleviate strain, worry, and tension. These calming oil blends are helpful in relieving both emotional and physical tension.

- Two or three drops of marjoram in a blend. This oil is a vasodilator that seems to lower high blood pressure by dilating arteries and small capillaries, allowing the blood to flow more easily.

- Two drops of oil of bergamot, whose key actions are relaxing and soporific, can influence blood pressure in a positive way.

- One drop of neroli, with its hypnotic properties, will help to soothe and calm down overwrought emotional states.

- Three drops of ylang-ylang are helpful to use when in need of relaxation, as this essence is excellent for high-strung, excitable conditions. This essential oil has the ability to regulate adrenaline, easing its flow. The euphoric, yet relaxing, aroma calms mental tension. This oil is an example of the adaptogenic qualities some essential oils have.

These essential oils can be blended in about 2 to 3 teaspoons (10 to 15 ml) of the carrier of your choice. A luxurious way to enjoy their aroma that helps you to de-stress and relax is bathing with a suitable essential oil.

Body massage is another way to use essential oils therapeutically when trying to lower high blood pressure. Simply rub the blended mixture in the palm of your hand to make sure it is evenly distributed. Apply it to the body using a massage technique.

Vaporizing oils is a way to create a perfumed ambience. Essence burners have a lower compartment for a candle and a small saucer on top, filled with water, into which a few drops of the oil are added. The heat from the candle evaporates the water and oil, releasing and vaporizing the aroma into the atmosphere.

A weekly aroma-massage is very relaxing and therapeutic for this condition, and it may bring blood pressure down to normal levels. This is a condition that can be related to high stress levels, so it may not even need drug therapy provided by a medical doctor.

Low Blood Pressure

This condition can be the result of a thyroid problem, and it must first be diagnosed by a medical doctor. Individuals prone to low blood pressure can experience dizziness and fainting due to interruption of the blood to the brain. The oils to use for low blood pressure are from the stimulating group. They can help rebalance the circulatory system and may help to elevate blood pressure. If you have a thyroid problem, do not stop any medication that has been prescribed without consulting a medical doctor.

- For a blend that can help elevate blood pressure, blend two drops of black pepper, with its warming aroma, with 2 teaspoons (10 ml) of your chosen carrier.

- Two drops of stimulating and restorative peppermint, blended with 2 teaspoons (10 ml) of a suitable base oil, can help to elevate blood pressure.

- Another blend that can be tried is two drops rosemary added to a base oil that helps the circulatory system. The fresh, green fragrance of this stimulating oil is ideal for use when the circulatory system is out of balance.

Daily baths using combinations of the above oils blended into a base are excellent for helping to improve the circulation of this condition and assisting low blood pressure. A stimulating aroma-massage will also prove therapeutic. Another way to help regulate this condition is to put rosemary in an essence burner so that you can inhale the flow of this stimulating oil.

Aroma Helpers: Sedatives for High BP clary sage, marjoram, and ylang-ylang

Aroma Helpers: Stimulators for Low BP peppermint, pine, and rosemary

The Dermatological System

The skin is the largest organ of the body and acts as a barrier between the body's internal organs and the environment. It consists of two main regions: the epidermis and the dermis. The epidermis is the outer layer that consists chiefly of dead, dry, flattened cells. These constantly shed and more cells are produced from the layer of living cells below the epidermis. This layer is called the dermis, a deeper layer, made up of living cells. The dermis performs a number of functions, but the two principal ones are absorption and elimination. The skin gets rid of waste products and toxins.

This system is prone to many ailments and needs a lot of care to keep it in good condition.

Acne

This distressing skin problem damages self-confidence. Acne is caused by the overproduction of oil from the sebaceous glands, combined with a bacterial infection. This skin condition can strike at any age, but is most common during puberty, when hormones become active and can become imbalanced, and it can also occur during menopause. Acne is most commonly found on the face, but the back and chest can also be affected, because these areas have a lot of sebaceous glands.

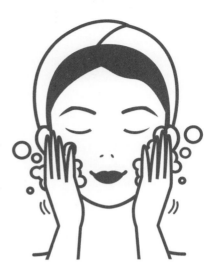

Acne can be helped by using essential oils. Most oils have antiseptic qualities that can help treat acne-prone skin, but good hygiene is vital to prevent constant recurrence of spots and pustules.

HIT THE SPOT WITH ESSENTIAL OILS

- Bergamot's balancing and antiseptic qualities are excellent for skin care, especially for blemished or oily skin. Use in a steam facial to cleanse the pores and heal the skin. Nonirritating in dilution, but can cause photosensitivity.
- Petitgrain, with its sharp, green, and orange-like aroma, can be used in a facial sauna for problems such as acne.
- Chamomile is an excellent oil to use in skin care due to its anti-inflammatory properties that help to relieve inflamed and itchy skin.
- Geranium's astringent qualities can clear toxins from the body, and its antiseptic action helps to control acne.
- Juniper is considered to be a toning and purifying oil that opens clogged pores and cleanses greasy, unhealthy skin.
- Lavender can be used neat on acne and any scars that may have resulted.
- Lemon, with its tangy, citrus fragrance, clarifies greasy skin and supports the liver, which is a detoxification organ. It is good for lymphatic cleansing. Use lemon blended with a base oil.
- Patchouli's astringent and antiseptic actions can aid in the treatment of oily skin and acne.
- Tea tree oil is a useful as an antibacterial and antifungal oil that is widely used for acne and blemish-prone skin. Tea tree oil helps reduce inflammation.

Add two drops of any of the above essential oils to 2 teaspoons (10 ml) of a light carrier, follow with a splash of skin lotion made from ten drops of calming lavender oil to 3.5 tablespoons (50 ml) of spring water to help heal acne. Dab individual pustules and spots with neat lavender or tea tree oil.

In nutritional medicine, it is believed that the skin acts as a third kidney. Acne, therefore, according to this theory, is linked to a system that is overloaded with toxins that the body is trying to clear, but which it has been unable to do via the normal channels of elimination.

Minor Skin Problems

For minor abrasions, scratches, mild burns, and stings, the therapeutic properties of the following oils are helpful:

Lavender: This popular oil can be used where there has been a cut, burn, or sting, due to its antibacterial properties. In the case of abrasions, scratches, and mild burns or stings, apply it neat as soon as possible to prevent infection.

Niaouli: This antibacterial oil, when mixed with carrier oil, will prevent infection on any minor skin condition.

Eucalyptus: Apply this antiseptic oil, mixed with a carrier, to soothe any of the above mild skin problems.

Boils and Abscesses These are infected pus-filled swellings. If large, they may need medical treatment to clear them up. They take a few days to develop, during which time they cause pain, inflammation, and tenderness. Hot compresses to "draw out the boil" made from lavender, tea tree, or eucalyptus oil will encourage the boil or abscess to open and to speed up healing. Niaouli's disinfectant action also helps, due to its antibacterial properties. Lemon or chamomile used in a hot compress can also be used. Add one drop of three of these oils to 7 tablespoons (100 ml) of hot water and use a clean piece of cotton, soaked in hot water. Wring this out and hold against the boil until the compress cools down. Repeat this several times a day. The heat will bring the boil to a head. Cleanse the surrounding area with neat tea tree oil and apply neat tea tree to the boil. When it opens, use lavender to cleanse and heal the wound. Treat the area daily with four drops of juniper and regular baths to detoxify the system, since boils and abscesses are a symptom of a system clogged with toxic wastes.

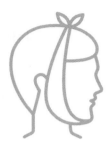

Tooth Abscess Use a cotton swab to apply some antiseptic clove oil on a painful tooth. This can provide some temporary relief from toothache, but severe pain is a sign that the tooth has developed an infection or an abscess, usually in the root area, and needs the attention of a dentist.

Cellulite This resembles dimpled, "orange peel" skin. It mainly affects women and seems related to female hormones. Cellulite forms on the upper arms, hips, buttocks, and thighs, and its distinctive, puckered, lumpy appearance can also appear on the stomach and knees. These nodules of fat are caused by poor circulation leading to a buildup of toxins and fluid due to poor elimination. Characterized by water retention and toxic wastes in the connective tissue surrounding the fat cells, cellulite is unattractive, so women spend fortunes on commercially produced creams in the hope that they will remove it. The tissue around these cells tends to harden causing the unsightly bumpy and uneven skin. Linked to lymphatic congestion as well as poor circulation, aromatherapy aims to stimulate the lymphatic system, balance the hormones, and reduce water retention. The following oils are suggested to help reduce fluid buildup. Cellulite is notoriously difficult to get rid of, but regular exfoliation, skin brushing with sea salt, and the addition of appropriate essential oils will at least effect some improvement.

Anti-Cellulite Oils The essential oils juniper, lavender, and lemongrass blended in a softening cold-pressed vegetable oil base, can be used on a regular basis. Massage firmly onto the skin concentrating on areas that are prone to cellulite. Massage encourages absorption of the oils into the epidermis, enhancing the cleansing effect, stimulating circulation, and helping to improve the appearance of this lumpy "orange peel" skin. Regular massage may be enhanced by the use of a massage mitten or loofah. This massage is most beneficial if used after a warm bath. Regular lymphatic massages and bathing, using cleansing essential oils—in particular, grapefruit with its diuretic properties—will help reduce fluid retention and cellulite. Perseverance should help clear up the condition, although it will take time, because cellulite is stubborn. At the same time, a cleansing diet should be followed.

Cypress, geranium, grapefruit, or lemon can also be tried in a synergistic blend in a light base oil.

Eczema Essential oils that are cleansing and anti-inflammatory, such as chamomile, geranium, and lavender, blended with 2 tablespoons (30 ml) of vegetable oil and applied to the affected area, can help to soothe this condition. Be cautious, however, as some people with eczema are allergic to all perfumes, even essential oils.

Psoriasis This skin problem is related to the immune system and is called an auto-immune disease. This occurs when the immune system goes into overdrive and attacks the body, or, in this case, the skin. Psoriasis is a mysterious condition that is not well understood by mainstream medicine. It seems to get worse with stress, can be in remission for a long time, and then flares up again. Alternative natural health practitioners and practitioners of nutritional medicine believe that this condition is related to a "leaky gut." Essential oils have been found to be helpful.

Psoriasis Blend Carrier oils—avocado or wheatgerm or evening primrose oil—with a few drops added of chamomile or bergamot to reduce inflammation, and juniper to improve circulation. Lavender can be added instead of one of these oils.

This blend may not work for everyone who suffers from psoriasis as it is a difficult skin problem that does not always respond well to creams, whether alternative or orthodox. It is a case of trial and error until the right mixture is found, but the therapeutic effect of aromatherapy oils is worth a try. When the correct blend for the individual who has the condition is found, improvements can occur, so do not give up.

Stretch Marks Although stretch marks are not a dermatological problem, they are unsightly and women do not like them. They can appear after weight loss, pregnancy, or teenage growth spurts. A massage blend made up of a carrier oil of your choice and the oils neroli and mandarin will help to heal even old stretch marks. For best results, apply once a day. Rose oil is good for stretch marks and scars.

Aroma Helpers: Balancing bergamot, geranium, and lavender

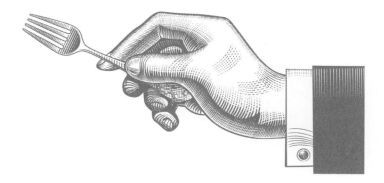

The Digestive System

The alimentary canal and the organs connected with it, such as the liver, are part of this important system. It is concerned with the intake and breakdown of food and needs to be in good working order for good health. This system can be prone to a number of uncomfortable problems such as indigestion, irritable bowel syndrome, heartburn, and a sluggish digestive system.

Indigestion can be caused by difficulty in digesting food and by eating food that is too spicy. Try to avoid this by eating foods with a milder flavor and drinking peppermint tea after a meal. A comfortable, relaxing setting when sitting down to eat and eating slowly help to avoid indigestion, as sometimes this is caused by tension and stress. Avoid eating late at night.

- Ginger, used in massage or diffusion, calms down the digestive system.
- Lemon is useful for stimulating the appetite. It tones the digestive system and is helpful for indigestion as well.
- Peppermint, known as a "digestive," is a well-known remedy for digestive disorders.
- Lavender helps digestive problems caused by stress, stomachache, and nausea.
- Massage the upper abdomen gently in a slow clockwise direction with a mixture of 6 tablespoons (90 ml) of a carrier oil to two drops of any one of the essential oils suggested.

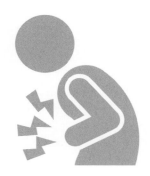

- Chamomile's soothing properties can help indigestion, colic, and peptic ulcers. Use as a warm compress, a massage over the painful area, or in a bath or diffusion.

Irritable Bowel Syndrome Peppermint oil is an antispasmodic and so will help to relieve the painful spasms caused by irritable bowel syndrome. This condition is not well understood, and some doctors do not even believe it exists. However, using peppermint oil mixed with chamomile and lavender, well diluted in a soothing massage over the abdominal area, will help to ease the painful spasms of this condition.

To get a sluggish digestive system moving, a blend of marjoram and geranium in a carrier oil massaged over the abdominal area will help stimulate and encourage a strong squeezing action of the muscular walls of the large intestine so that it does its job of moving waste material.

Aroma Helpers: Soothers peppermint, orange, and mandarin

The Endocrine System

A number of separate ductless glands are involved in the human glandular system known as the endocrine system. This system is concerned with controlling the body's general activities, which include the growth and development of the body. Involved with hormone production, the glands secrete chemical messengers into the bloodstream and lymphatic system. The body can be kept in a state of good health only if the hormones needed to stimulate a particular activity are in balance. We live in a stressful environment these days, and these glands can get out of balance. Stress has become the "modern" disease.

Aromatherapy has some very good oils that can help to reinstate homeostasis, or bring a system back into balance. These oils have the remarkable property that they can be stimulating and calming at the same time. Known as adaptogens or balancers, these oils assist us to adapt to stressors through their ability to restore equilibrium. Mother Nature has many herbal adaptogens and plant oil adaptogens as well. When used, they attune to the body's requirements. Used in combination, their healing abilities are strengthened.

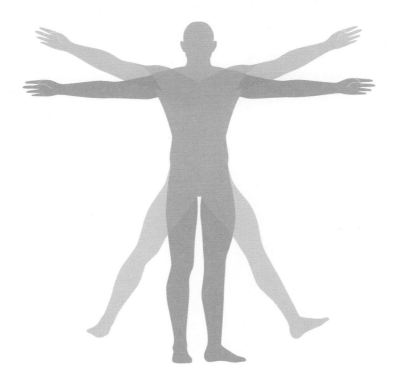

Stressful conditions, anxiety, panic attacks, constant worry, and so on will put your hormones into overdrive, flooding the body with stress hormones. This constant stress overload is very damaging and can lead to serious health problems. Continual stress has been known to activate dormant genes that bring on diseases that may be in your genetic patterns, but would otherwise have remained inactive. If you do not learn to "switch off," these stressful hormones can trigger these ailments into activity. It is therefore important to keep this glandular system healthy. Overfunctioning glands need to be encouraged to revert to a homeostatic state. Underfunctioning glands need stimulation to bring them back into equilibrium. This is where the adaptogenic oils come into their element.

I cannot say that these oils have been proven scientifically to act in this way, but many aromatherapy practitioners have found this to be so. There is still a lot that is not understood about the way essential oils work, but we do know they work, through empirical evidence and observation over thousands of years.

If there are any hormonal imbalances in either under-functioning or over-functioning glands, these healing balancers can be used with therapeutic effect:

Basil: This is useful for over-functioning hormones, nervous insomnia, and mental strain. Stressed-out states increase cortisol, the stress hormone. Basil's balancing effect increases the body's natural response to these situations helping the body's hormonal systems to cope in a better way. *Adaptogenic*

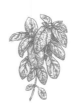

Clary sage: Over-functioning hormones and high blood pressure due to nervous tension can be calmed with this oil, enabling the body to reinstate the correct balance needed to promote good health. *Adaptogenic*

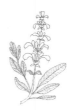

Geranium: This homeostatic oil will help to calm an overwrought system, improving hormonal function when tension has caused restlessness, panic attacks, and anxiety. *Adaptogenic*

Lavender: Reactions to stress, such as palpitations, high blood pressure, and irritability will respond well to the calming and restorative effect of this healing oil. *Adaptogenic*

Lemon: This oil's stimulating fragrance will help underfunctioning hormones reinstate the correct balance, enabling the body to function in a healthier way. *Adaptogenic*

Lemongrass: This strengthening oil relieves depression, tension, and nervous exhaustion—all signs that the hormones are overfunctioning and need calming down. *Adaptogenic*

Ylang-ylang: This is a balancer that will calm frayed nerves, and it is also a relaxant. A few drops on a handkerchief inhaled deeply will be beneficial to someone who has low blood pressure. It will also help nervous or emotional people who tend to get palpitations. Put into a warm bath, it is useful as a relaxant. This oil does not share the adaptogenic qualities of some other oils, but it has a balancing, sedating, and relaxing effect on the emotions.

Physical reactions to stress are usually a sign that the adrenal glands are overworked. Positioned across the upper end of each kidney, these glands produce the stress hormone cortisol and many other hormones. Calming hormone output from these glands is important, and therapeutic oils used in healing massage, baths, diffusers, and inhalations can do this.

Insomnia

Lack of sleep can be very wearing and may be the result of stress-related anxiety and nervous tension. Worry over the day's events can also result in sleepless nights. The use of the sedative herbs below can help soothe an overactive mind, thereby promoting restful sleep.

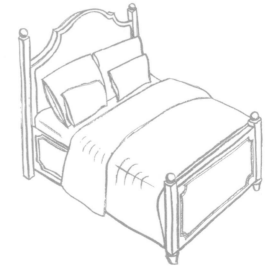

Aroma Helpers: Sedatives, proven natural sleep aids and stress-reducers in aromatherapy's armory, are lavender, cypress, chamomile, and melissa

Aroma Helpers: Energizers lemon, orange, and grapefruit to stimulate the glands

The Immune System

This vital system is critically important and should be kept in good condition in order to help you withstand viral and bacterial attacks. A healthy and well-functioning immune system will keep disease-causing materials from entering your body. If the barriers of this system fail, any number of diseases can result, from external influences and also if an imbalance occurs within the body, whereby the immune system attacks the body, resulting in auto-immune diseases such as rheumatoid arthritis, allergies, and so forth. To avoid this serious malfunction, there are immune-boosting essential oils that you can use.

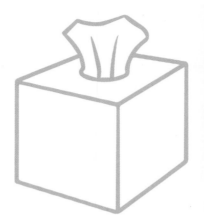

Scientific studies show that emotional and physiological stress impacts this sensitive system negatively. Oils that help to build up a system weakened by stress, overuse of drugs, and poor nutrition are bergamot, Roman chamomile, lavender, and myrrh. These oils, diluted in a carrier, can be applied on the neck and the temples. They can also be used in baths, inhalations, and diffusers.

Other oils that have immune-boosting properties are eucalyptus, lemongrass, ravensara, rosemary, and thyme. They encourage the production of white blood cells by activating them so that they collect in the areas where the bacteria or viruses are multiplying. This enables the immune system to fight off these disease-carrying germs.

Allergies

During the annual pollen season, many people suffer from hay fever, which is an allergic response to trees, weeds, grasses, shrubs, and farm crops. Allergies are an immune response to a harmful allergen, whereby the immune system overreacts, so calming this system down will help ameliorate these seasonal allergies. Hay-fever symptoms include allergic rhinitis, frequent sneezing, itchy, watery eyes, and inflammation of the nose and throat caused by airborne irritants.

When a warm day follows a period of cold and dampness, there is a buildup of pollen in the plants. In the country, exposure to pollen occurs in the late evening, whereas in the city, this happens from late evening to late at night. It is not always easy to avoid going out at these times. With the use of aromatherapy oils *before* the pollen season starts, you may be able to lessen the symptoms of these distressing allergies.

Cedarwood: This soothing oil can help relieve the mucus congestion and sinusitis of hay fever. Try it in a steam inhalation.

Chamomile: The anti-inflammatory properties of this oil can help control the inflammatory response of the immune system in allergic reactions. Three drops of chamomile mixed with one drop of eucalyptus in a room burner will create a calming atmosphere that is beneficial for allergic conditions. The same blend can also be used for sinusitis in 2 teaspoons (10 ml) of carrier oil, to massage the sinuses. Eucalyptus: This oil can relieve the symptoms of hay fever when used in a relaxing bath. Its decongestant properties work well used as a massage oil mixed with a light carrier. A drop or two on your pillow at night will help you to breathe more easily and get a good night's sleep. During the day, carry a handkerchief with one or two drops of eucalyptus and sniff it regularly to keep your airways clear.

Frankincense: Make up a massage blend with this anti-inflammatory oil and rub it onto the chest to relieve congestion in the case of hay fever. Try it in the bath as a stress-reliever.

Juniper: This oil helps to tone up the glandular system and, when used in a diffuser, can purify and detox the air during the allergy season.

Aroma Helpers: Immune Boosters tea tree, rosemary, lemon, geranium, and eucalyptus

The Limbic System

The primitive brain is based in a series of parts known as the limbic system. The sense of smell is connected to this area of the brain. We all have an emotional and instinctive reaction to aromas, so we either love a smell or recoil from it. Through the use of the sense of smell we can uplift our emotions, feel better, and gain a more optimistic view of life. Every time we inhale a heavenly smelling perfume or essential oil, we benefit from the experience. The sense of smell is more important than people are aware of, and while

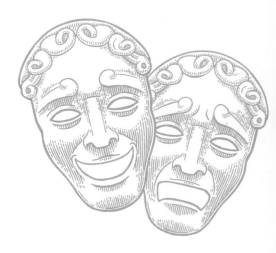

ancient civilizations appear to have known this and made use of its benefits, modern medicine does not seem to acknowledge this. Happily, the age-old practice of aromatherapy can address this omission. The best way to improve well-being if you are feeling low is to choose any of the oils that appeal to you the most.

Clary sage: Used in a burner to scent the air, this oil can lift depression, calm the emotions, and enhance feelings of well-being.

Bergamot: This oil has an antidepressant effect and helps to uplift the mood. Use a few drops in a hot diffuser. A candle or electricity heats the oil and water prevents overheating.

Aroma Helpers: Antidepressants basil, cedarwood, and lemongrass

The Lymphatic System

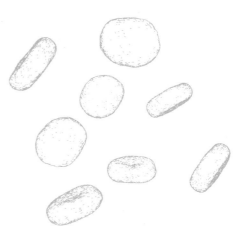

This system contains lymph, a watery fluid that originates in the spaces between cells. Lymph drains into networks of tiny capillaries in tissue spaces that unite to form larger vessels called lymphatics. This important network is part of the immune system. It is the main way that the body is protected from microorganisms, and keeping the lymphatic fluids healthy will go a long way toward preventing illness. Unlike the heart, which pumps blood throughout the body, this system does not have such a mechanism, and it can often become congested and sluggish. It is important to keep the watery fluid of the lymphatics moving, clearing toxic wastes. Regular skin brushing and the use of decongesting oils are ways to get the lymphatic fluids moving throughout the body in order to eliminate toxic wastes.

Peppermint oil: This anti-inflammatory oil cleanses the lymphatic system. In a massage blend, add five drops of peppermint oil to 2 teaspoons (10 ml) of a blending oil of your choice. Make sure that a body massage with this oil uses well-diluted peppermint, as the smell is strong. Other than these cautions, an invigorating shower with this cooling oil will help aid waste removal. Sprinkle a few drops on a flannel or a washcloth. Do not use if skin is sensitive or in concentrations over 3 percent.

Caution Not suitable for young children.

Aroma Helpers: Stimulators to Aid Circulation juniper, ginger, and rosemary

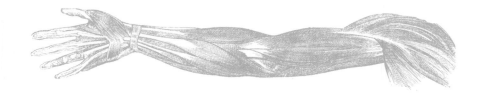

The Musculoskeletal System

The muscular system forms the flesh of the body and provides the means by which we carry out all forms of movement. The skeletal system, made up of bone, supports and protects the body, giving it shape.

Activity Injuries Certain activities, vigorous sports, for example, can put a strain on the joints. The essential oils of lavender, rosemary, marjoram, and vetiver help relieve the pain and tenderness of torn or damaged ligaments. But do not massage a sprain as this could make it worse. Use a cold compress with any one of these oils and keep the joint rested. You can also add two drops of the oil of your choice to 2 teaspoons (10 ml) fragrance-free lotion and apply to the area when the pain and swelling in the joint has reduced.

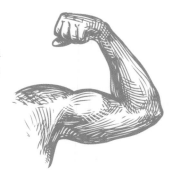

Back Pain This is a very common ailment and thousands of days are taken off because of it. Back pain can become very severe and chronic. There are a number of aromatherapy oils that can help this debilitating condition. These are soothing chamomile, warming black pepper, relaxing lavender, and sweet marjoram, useful for aching back muscles. You can take a warm bath in which you have put a few drops of essential oil or make a warm compress. A back massage is very

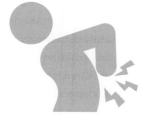

therapeutic at this time and may ease the pain.

Preventing Muscular Aches Warming massage balm using a carrier oil containing soothing lavender and penetrating black pepper oil can be used as a muscle rub before any type of exercise to help prevent muscle strain.

Muscular Aches If you still experience general aches and muscular pains after exercise, or any other muscle pain, the essential oils of basil for its restorative properties, warming, relaxing marjoram, and toning rosemary can be used to soothe your aching muscles. Make up a massage blend with 2 teaspoons (10 ml) of a carrier oil and a few drops of the essential oil of your choice—or a mixture, for example: one drop of basil, two drops of rosemary, and two drops of marjoram. Massage the area daily with this potent blend of healing oils until the aches or pains are relieved. If you prefer, these oils can be used individually.

Osteoarthritis This painful degenerative joint disease is the most common form of arthritis, affecting many middle-aged and elderly people. Women are twice as likely to suffer from it as men. Sedentary lifestyles can be a contributing factor. Many people suffer from painful osteoarthritis of the knee, necessitating surgery for knee replacements; unfortunately, these are not always successful.

The painful joints due to wear and tear can be gently massaged around the sore areas using a carrier oil with essential oils of eucalyptus, rosemary, and juniper.

Osteoporosis This is a loss of bone tissue. The bones become increasingly porous and brittle and can fracture very easily. This condition is more common in women. Oils that may help bone repair are cypress, frankincense, and rosewood. These can be used in a therapeutic massage treatment and applied topically. Gently massage the painful areas, being careful not to exert too much pressure.

Both osteoarthritis and osteoporosis benefit from the use of oils with analgesic and vasodilatory qualities such as lavender, juniper, ginger, and marjoram. A few drops of your chosen oil, blended with a carrier, in a warm bath will help detoxify the system and ease aches and pains.

Aroma Helpers: Sedatives clary sage, chamomile, orange, bergamot

The Nervous System

The brain and spinal cord form the central nervous system. This system provides the means by which we can respond to stimuli, and it controls muscles, endocrine glands, and so on. It is a complicated structure that is prone to tension, stress, and anxiety. Long-term stress can unbalance this delicate system, resulting in physical disease, high blood pressure, skin problems, and mood disorders. Luckily, aromatherapy can come to the rescue. Geranium oil helps to restore emotional harmony when nerves are frayed. Other oils have therapeutic value in treating conditions related to the central nervous system, such as soothing, cooling chamomile, with its ability to calm irritability and nervousness, and mandarin, a comforting oil that gently calms the nerves.

Migraine This debilitating and painful condition afflicts many people. Add

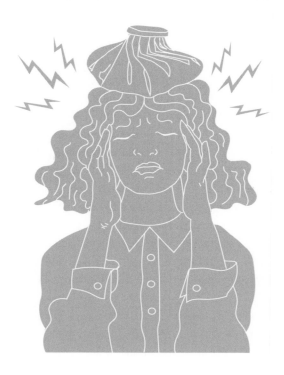

a suitable essential oil—Roman chamomile, lemon balm, lavender, sweet marjoram, peppermint, and clary sage all work well—to a damp washcloth and place this on the forehead as a cool compress. Use ice-cold water with four to five drops of the essential oil of your choice; dip in a cloth and wring it out. Place it on the forehead or the back of the neck. This may ease the headache and nausea brought on by this condition. Try to prevent an attack, but do not give treatment during one, as this condition tends to make people hypersensitive, and use of the oils may cause a reaction. Migraine sufferers usually know the symptoms of an impending attack.

Aroma Helpers: Soothers clary sage and rosemary

Neuralgia This condition is caused by pain arising along the course of a nerve, and the pain can be stabbing, dull, or severe. It can be triggered by a nerve becoming irritated or compressed, or there may be inflammation or

MOOD AND EMOTIONAL BALANCERS

Aromatherapy has many oils that can help bring frazzled emotions back into a harmonious and balanced state. There are essences that can uplift, refresh, and relax. If an emotional boost is required, there are suitable oils to help energize a flagging system. Pick some plant oils from nature's garden, mix them in a suitable carrier to create a blend that can promote a number of positive states, and enjoy their de-stressing benefits. Put a few drops into a bowl of water and place near a source of heat to fill the air with their wonderful fragrance. Alternatively, use a light bulb ring or essential oil burner to vaporize the oil.

The oils listed below will help to create a mood-enhancing atmosphere, relieving a low mood and calming anxious thoughts and nervous exhaustion.

- Refreshing: pine, lemon, peppermint, eucalyptus

- Relaxing: clary sage, chamomile, lavender, neroli, sandalwood

- Energizing: ginger, juniper, peppermint, pine, rosemary

- Calming: chamomile, lavender, lemon balm, myrrh

infection present. Facial neuralgia can be set off by cold wind. This painful and debilitating condition is also aggravated by stress. Roman chamomile, eucalyptus, and marjoram are powerful analgesic and nervine oils that can be used to ease the pain.

You can make a massage blend of any of the above essential oils. Or you can make a hot compress and place it over the affected part. Put drops into a diffuser or sprinkle a few drops in a stress-releasing bath.

Aroma Helpers geranium and thyme

Shingles This very painful nerve condition is caused by the herpes zoster virus that is also responsible for chicken pox. This virus lies hidden in the body, and at times when the immune system is weakened, usually as a result of emotional stress or age, it can reactivate and manifest as a blistering rash that normally occurs around one half of the midriff. The eyes, face, and neck can also be affected, as a result of inflamed nerve roots. Baths are the easiest way to treat shingles. These oils have been found to help ease the nerve pain of this extremely painful condition:

Geranium: Its cooling and moisturizing properties, mixed with thyme oil in a base, will help to strengthen the immune response. This combination will create a healing mixture that can be dabbed gently onto the affected area. It is more helpful if this mixture is used at the first sign of a rash.

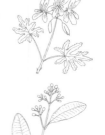

Ravensara: Used for treating viral infections, this oil is a good rubbing oil for shingles. Ravensara's warming action, blended with thyme—another warming oil—will create a potent healing mix that can help alleviate the acute pain of this condition.

Any irritated nerves, including sciatica, can also be treated using nervines. Powerful analgesic and nervine oils are required to relieve the nerve pain caused by these conditions. Such oils are known to exert a soothing effect along the nerve pathways and are the "three stars" of the nervine group, offering some much-needed pain relief:

Aroma Helpers: Pain Relievers Chamomile soothes sciatica and nerve irritation; marjoram has analgesic properties and is a good pain reliever.

The Reproductive System

This system consists of different organs in the male and female. It is concerned with the formation of cells involved in reproduction, the ovum and the sperm. This is an area in both women and men that needs care in order to prevent problems.

Female System

The female reproductive organs are prone to a number of problems, and orthodox medicine has a special branch that deals with all female problems.

Endometriosis This is a poorly understood condition that causes pain and infertility. It is caused by tissue that normally lines the inside of the uterus growing outside this organ. This tissue attaches to the pelvis, bladder, colon, and ovaries causing pain every month during the menstrual cycle. Endometriosis is not well understood by mainstream medicine but is believed to be caused by hormonal imbalances, genetics, or even stress.

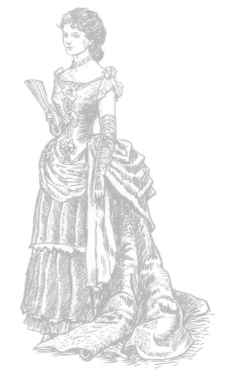

Clary sage is a hormone balancer that can be effective in reducing symptoms. For a massage blend, use two to four drops and 6 tablespoons (90 ml) carrier oil; apply topically over the abdomen. Another way to reduce symptoms is to apply a warm compress over the abdominal area during the menstrual cycle, particularly when the pain is most acute. Two other oils with hormone-balancing properties are rose and geranium, and either would be useful to try.

Irregular Periods When the cycle has an irregular pattern, and if periods are delayed, cedarwood can stimulate late periods. Regular aromatherapy treatment with soothing oils can bring the menstrual cycle back to normal. A blend of chamomile, melissa, and rose is a known regulator of the menstrual flow.

Period Pains and Cramps Many women experience painful cramps during their periods, and the intensity of the pain can vary from month to month. Unless there is an underlying problem that needs medical attention, the aromatherapy oils cypress, clary sage, and jasmine can reduce uterine cramps.

Aroma Helpers: Balancers Lavender, rosemary, and marjoram

Male System

The prostate gland is the size of a chestnut and is situated just below the bladder. There are several aroma essences that can be rubbed into the abdomen to maintain overall prostate health.

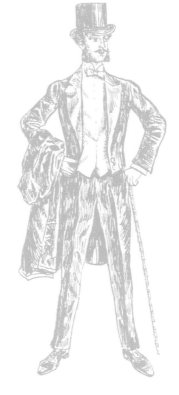

- Frankincense supports prostate health due to its anti-inflammatory properties. Blended with strengthening myrrh and cooling geranium and used as a massage with a base oil of your choice, or as a compress or bath, frankincense can help if you are experiencing discomfort.

- Juniper berry oil has warming, stimulating, and toning action that supports urinary and prostate health.

- Prostatitis is inflammation of this gland, which can lead to urinary problems. This condition needs a visit to your doctor. However, frankincense and cleansing thyme in a base oil used in therapeutic baths, massage, or compress, may help relieve symptoms. Keep in mind, though, that prostate problems can have serious underlying causes, so a visit to a medical doctor would be advisable.

Aroma Helpers: Sedatives Orange and myrtle

The Respiratory System

This system involves the exchange of gases (carbon dioxide and oxygen) between the blood and air. The trachea, the tube that connects the pharynx and larynx to the lungs, is part of this system. This area of the body can be easily damaged by smoking and environmental factors. Since it is prone to chest infections, asthma, allergies, and some serious diseases caused by smoking or inhalation of chemicals, this system needs looking after carefully. Aromatherapy offers ways that this can be done with regular use of essential oils.

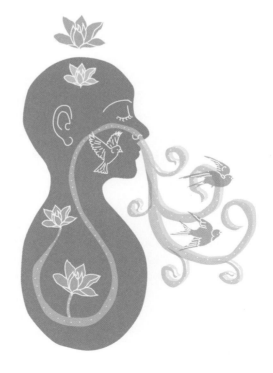

Bronchitis Benzoin plus eucalyptus in a cream or carrier oil used as a chest rub can help free chest mucus. These are known as expectorants, which liquefy bronchial secretions.

Chest Colds The same blend used to treat the symptoms of bronchitis can be used to free up the chest mucus that comes with chest colds. An aromatic chest rub made up of eucalyptus, rosemary, and tea tree oils in a base will help to soothe and ease minor coughs, colds, and stuffy noses. Apply this to the thoracic area daily. Keep in mind that peppermint's strong smell may cause a headache in those who are susceptible. Otherwise, peppermint's expectorant qualities help coughs that produce green or yellow phlegm, which are signs of infection.

Sinusitis Inhalations through aromatic steam are helpful for this condition. Eucalyptus with its decongestant properties, along with peppermint, are ideal oils to use to help relieve a stuffy nose and sinusitis.

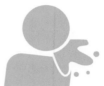

An inhalation made up of niaouli with its strong camphorous aroma, and basil with its clearing properties, makes this an ideal blend with unique cleansing and decongesting abilities, helping to clear and maintain healthy sinuses. This mixture can also be used in an oil burner so that the vapors diffuse in the air.

Aroma Helpers: Cleansers Eucalyptus, lemon, tea tree, and rosemary

The Urinary System

The kidneys and associated structures are part of the urinary system. They are involved in the removal of waste material in liquid form and also with keeping the body in a state of balance. The female urinary system is more prone to infections than the male system due to its anatomical structure.

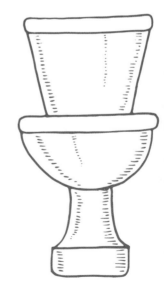

Cystitis This is caused by an infection in the urinary tract that women are more prone to than men. The symptoms are pain and frequency when urinating. Tea tree and sandalwood are oils that can be used with a hot compress applied to the abdominal area. Both have antiseptic properties. These oils can also be used in a bath, so bathe twice a day until the pain and burning has ceased.

Along with this treatment, drink plenty of pure water and unsweetened cranberry juice. If there is no improvement, consult a medical doctor.

A quick fix for cystitis is to drink a glass of water in which a half-teaspoon of sodium bicarbonate (baking powder) has been dissolved.

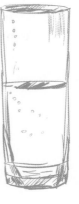

Aroma Helpers: Toners Cedarwood, geranium, and juniper

❀ ❀ ❀

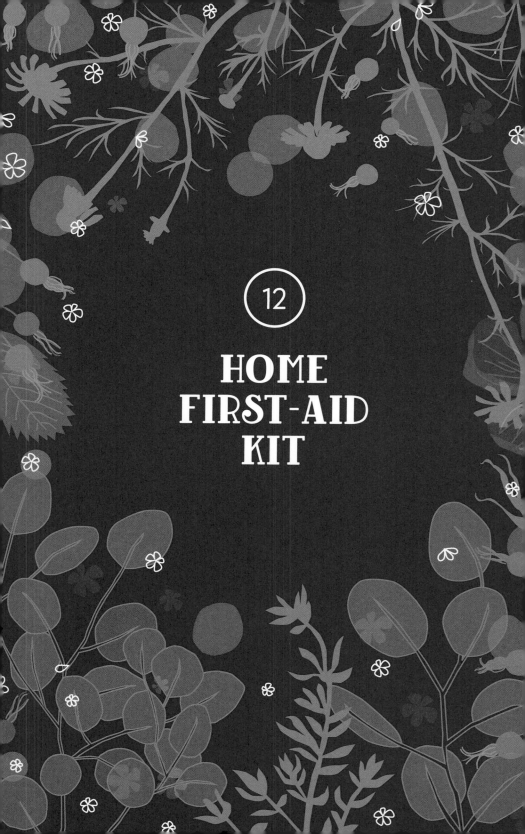

12

HOME
FIRST-AID
KIT

"Aromatherapy is the skilled and controlled use of essential oils for physical and emotional health and wellbeing."

Valerie Cooksley

There are so many oils to choose from for a home first-aid kit that, for a novice, this can be somewhat daunting. I suggest some of the oils that are easy to obtain, as many are not available to the public, but only to professional aromatherapists. Always buy your essential oils from a good supplier, as they can vary in quality, and keep in mind that only the best will act therapeutically. You can gradually build a home collection of aromatherapy oils as you become more experienced in their use. I have suggested ten easily obtainable oils to start you off. These everyday oils, kept in your home, will provide you with natural health care on a day-to-day basis, allowing you to act swiftly for any minor problem that occurs.

Your first-aid kit will contain oils that help colds, headaches, sinusitis, insomnia, muscle aches and pains, stress, insect bites, and minor abrasions—any condition, in fact, that is suitable for self-help.

Choose a few carrier oils to put in your home first-aid kit for therapeutic blending.

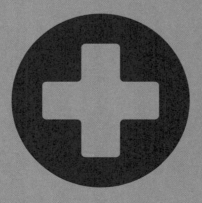

The Ten Healers

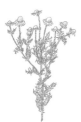

1. Chamomile Oil

This gentle oil is useful for indigestion, irritability, and painful attacks of neuralgia or sciatica, all treatable by self-help.

2. Eucalyptus Oil

This is helpful to use for headaches, muscle and joint aches, and insect bites.

3. Geranium Oil

This emotional healer is calming during times of stress and anxiety. It helps mild gastroenteritis and is useful for relieving menopausal symptoms. It is also a good insect repellent.

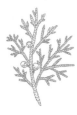

4. Juniper Berry Oil

Muscle pains brought on by cold weather can be eased with juniper's warming and toning action.

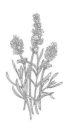

5. Lavender Oil

This highly versatile oil, which is almost a cure-all, can treat minor digestive problems that have a nervous origin and also nausea. Its mild analgesic properties make it a good first-aid remedy for headaches and also for abrasions, cuts, burns, stings, and insect bites.

6. Lemon Oil

During the winter, this oil will stimulate the body's defenses if used regularly, helping to prevent bacterial and viral infections. This is becoming very important now that resistance to antibiotics is on the rise. Lemon oil is also good for corns, verrucas, and warts.

7. Peppermint Oil

This cooling oil is well known to be effective for digestive disorders and stomachaches and is also useful for relieving stiffness in shoulders and joints. Its cooling properties are helpful in bringing down fevers.

8. Ravensara Oil

An antibacterial powerhouse, this oil is useful during the cold and flu season. Its pain-relieving action on muscles and joints has a relaxing effect.

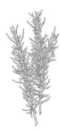

9. Rosemary

This reviving and invigorating oil reenergizes tired muscles and weary feet. Good for women's health, rosemary oil helps relieve painful periods.

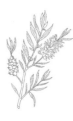

10. Tea Tree Oil

This potent antiseptic oil forms part of every aromatherapist's first-aid kit. Useful for general infections, tea tree also treats nailbed infections due to its antifungal properties, along with cuts, mild burns, and cold sores. Blended with lavender, this synergistic mixture offers relief from itching.

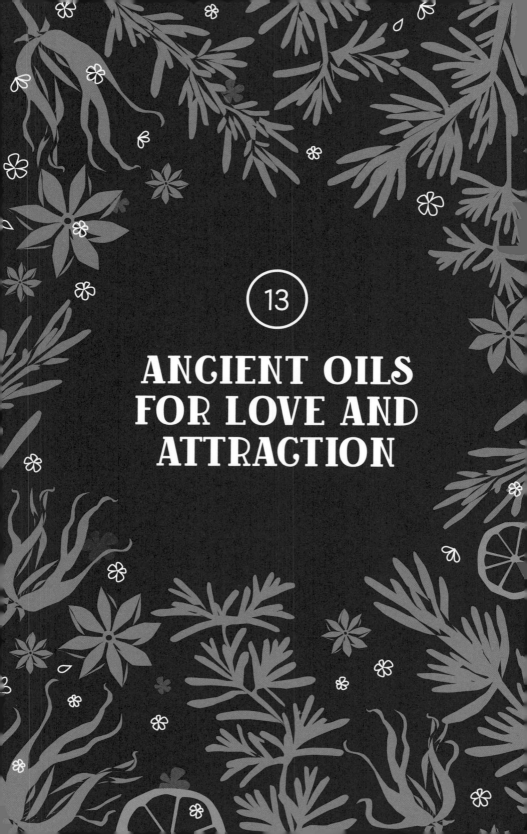

13

ANCIENT OILS FOR LOVE AND ATTRACTION

"I have perfumed my bed with myrrh, aloes,
and cinnamon."

The Book of Proverbs

Nature's cornucopia of oils can uplift you, invigorate your senses, and calm your soul. They can also act as an aphrodisiac, heightening passion and sexual desire. Ancient civilizations knew the power of these wonderful oils and how fragrance can enhance the senses. They have been used for centuries to attract the opposite sex. Used in the armory of seduction, they were potent weapons to use in the art of love. The canny ancient Egyptians, Greeks, and Romans knew that aromatherapy oils and their arousing aromas can improve your love life!

Aroma plays a fundamental role in human sexual response, which is why perfumes made with essential oils have been used for thousands of years and are still so popular today. The perfume industry is a multimillion-dollar business, and it knows how to exploit our love of fragrant aromas. The big perfume houses know that aroma—and the implication that a particular perfume will make you sexier and more attractive—sells. They know that our sense of smell is related to our emotions, moods, and sexual behavior, and that these areas can be stimulated through our sense of smell, linked to the primitive brain—the limbic system. The link between hormones and sexuality has been proven, and it appears that our sense of smell has developed for sensual purposes through the evolutionary process, as humans no longer need to "smell danger." A beautiful fragrance can influence the deep emotional part of us, evoking memories, uplifting us, and filling us with pleasure. Everyone has a different fragrance to which they respond, and each oil smells different from one person to another.

The beautiful Greek goddess Aphrodite, goddess of love, beauty, desire, and sexuality, gave us the word *aphrodisiac*. Her son Eros, god of love, passion, and fertility, gave us the word *erotic*, meaning "sexual love." Aphrodite was a seductress no man could resist. She was knowledgeable and skilled in the art of using aromatic plants for sexual purposes, and that gave her an advantage over her rivals. She not only used her beauty—she had the help of a collection of magical oils as well! Like the goddess herself, you can use the sorcery of sensual scents to captivate your lover!

Cleopatra, Queen of the Nile, met her new lover, Mark Antony, for the first time when she sailed down the River Nile with the purple sails of her flotilla of ships saturated in a heady mixture, believed today to have been a blend of rose and neroli, two powerful seductive essences. Redolent with the exotic, powerful, floral perfume of these seductive oils filling the air, Cleopatra would have been irresistible!

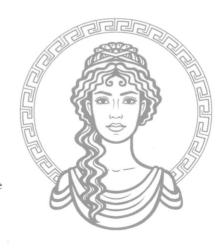

No wonder the ancient Egyptians, Greeks, and Romans were such keen users of these wonderful oils! They knew the power the oils had to stimulate desire and inflame the passions. Known for their decadence, the Romans used them abundantly for pleasure and for their aphrodisiac qualities.

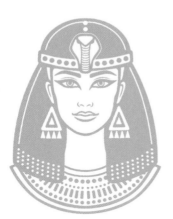

It was not only the ancient Egyptians, Greeks, and Romans who utilized the power of these essential oils. A manual of erotic arts titled *The Perfumed Garden*, written in the fourteenth century by a Tunisian sheik named Nefwazi, is the story of a man's use of perfumes and aromas to seduce the woman he loved.

Every partnership needs a boost now and again, and essential oils are renowned for having potent qualities that have the ability to excite the senses. Certain essential oils awaken and increase sexual desire. I have listed some below. Use them in the bedroom and find out for yourself! My list is only a suggestion, so you might, in time, come up with a list of your own.

Use the essential oils of your choice in a blend for sensual, erotic massage. Sensual baths can be created by adding a few drops of any one of the oils mentioned below.

Cedarwood Oil

The amazing, warm, woody, balsamic aroma can be very exciting. This is a good oil to use if you want to attract a new partner and keep the attraction alive. In an erotic encounter, it will make you feel warm and sexy and it will stir your passions.

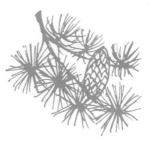

Clary Sage Oil

This hormone-balancing oil acts as a powerful aphrodisiac. It can clear any fears and negativity that may have affected a relationship. With its captivating fragrance, this oil can help set the mood for an improved and revitalized relationship.

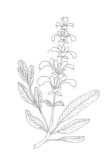

Geranium Oil

This oil helps to harmonize the emotions and it opens the heart chakra, enabling you to receive love. Pour three or four drops of essential oil in a little water in a perfume burner to have a flow filling the air.

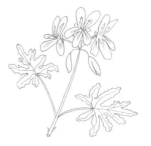

Tip

The chakras are an ancient system of sensitive points on the body that play a part in our health, psychology, feelings, and spirituality.

Jasmine Oil

One of the most expensive essences, jasmine oil is floral, exquisitely rich, and intoxicating. It stimulates the spirit as well as the physical senses. Working on an emotional level, this oil relaxes frayed nerves, calming the emotions so that desire will begin to flow.

Neroli Oil

This heady orange blossom perfume creates a warm and romantic atmosphere conducive to love and seduction. It has been used for centuries as a natural aphrodisiac.

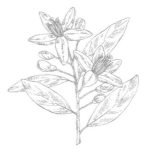

Patchouli Oil

During the flower-power era of the 1960s, "Make Love Not War" was the hippies' mantra. Embracing a natural lifestyle, hippies dropped out of mainstream society and created "free love." This arousing oil was one they used lavishly. Patchouli has a relaxing, sensual, exotic aroma with romantic overtones. It can evoke past memories that are shared by lovers, and its relaxing properties will get you and your partner in the right mood for love. It has a relaxing effect on the central nervous system, helping you to unwind.

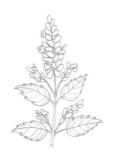

Rose Otto Oil

The queen of essential oils is the archetypal fragrance of love. This is the most romantic of all oils, as it stirs desire and sets the tone for a romantic encounter, preparing the heart chakra to receive love. This erotic fragrance has been used by lovers for millennia.

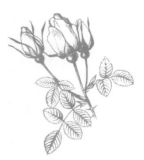

Vanilla Oil

A fragranced aphrodisiac used in burners and diffusers, vanilla oil will release its aroma to create a romantic atmosphere when you and your partner wish to enjoy passionate moments together.

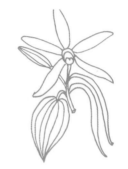

Ylang-Ylang Oil

This oil stimulates the passions of love and desire. Its floral essence will get you in the mood for love, working to arouse positive emotions and creating the right emotional and mental state for a passionate encounter.

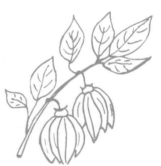

Aromatherapy massage is perfect for a sensual experience. A massage indulges two of our most important senses at the same time, these being touch and smell. Prepare blended massage oil from fragrant essential oils of your choice. I have only given some suggestions that will meet your wishes to create a sensual love potion, because everyone has different ideas about what smells good.

The feminine fragrances of rose, neroli, ylang-ylang, and jasmine are beautiful aromas for women, but men must not be left out. Masculine essential oils are cypress, sandalwood, vetiver, clary sage, and ylang-ylang. Any of these lovely, sensual, perfumed aromatherapy oils can be used to blend into love potions. Be as adventurous and daring as you want to be!

Love Potions

Using a carrier oil to create a sensual massage oil to use as a love potion, using a carrier oil, is an art in itself. Rose, a deeply feminine aroma, is a universal symbol of true love. This sweet and heady fragrance is certainly one to be used in any romantic blend. Vanilla is said to have aphrodisiac qualities and is wonderfully relaxing when used in a burner or diffuser; this oil has a lovely balsamic fragrance that will perfume the air and help a flagging libido!

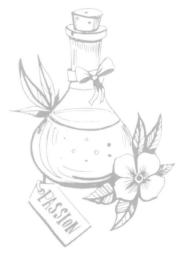

Using an aroma-touch massage technique that relaxes the whole body will help to create the right mood. Experiment with different combinations, using these voluptuous oils in blends. You can also use any oil with aphrodisiac properties to make a luxurious bath.

We all have different tastes when it comes to aromas, so go ahead and experiment, and when you have found your favorite scent, use it to create love potions of your own. Then see if they work!

Love Potion No. 1

For a sensual bath before a romantic tryst, use one drop each of rose, jasmine, and neroli, blended in 2 teaspoons (10 ml) of apricot-kernel oil. Let the oils seep into your skin to stimulate and restore your emotions. An erotic massage blend made with the oils of rosewood, energizing pine, and warming, relaxing clary sage is ideal to use when energy blocks have dampened emotions. This could be because of stress and anxiety. The combination of an uplifting fragrance with a therapeutic massage may help to stimulate desire.

Love Potion No.2

For a relaxing massage blend using aphrodisiac oils, you can try a combination of two drops of sensual ylang-ylang and one drop of restorative and relaxing sandalwood in 2 teaspoons (10 ml) of a base oil of your choice. This potion is a good choice if you want to stimulate a male partner's interest, as sandalwood's aphrodisiac qualities can help to increase libido in men. A massage with these fragrant oils not only will stir your emotions but you will also have wonderfully soft skin after this massage, and so will your partner. You can use a blend made up of 3 tablespoons (45 ml) carrier oil with two drops of sandalwood if you prefer.

Love Potion No.3

For a sensual blend, use the pure essential oils of patchouli, an oil that is known to increase libido; and sweet, musky ylang-ylang; and neroli, with its warm, floral undertones, in a sweet almond and vitamin E base oil. Let the aromas of this pleasurable blend waft around you as you enjoy its scented fragrance. This blend is ultra-relaxing and its sensual properties will work their magic, bringing a feeling of peace and balance, and putting you in a romantic mood. Bergamot, although less sensual, can also be used in a blend for an amorous meeting, as its deliciously orange-scented mood-enhancing fragrance stirs the senses.

Nights of Passion Blend

Mix this wonderful aphrodisiac blend for you and your partner:
- 1 drop of rose, with its warm, floral fragrance, to uplift the spirits.
- 1 drop of jasmine's exquisitely heady, sensuous fragrance to help create a spellbinding blend.
- 1 drop of sandalwood, with its distinctive, seductive tones, to set the mood.
    Blend them in a suitable carrier of your choice that will create the atmosphere . . . and let the magic begin!

14
MAGICAL BLENDS

*"Wind-bit thyme that smells like the perfume of
the dawn in Paradise."*

Rudyard Kipling

Blending essential oils is a fine art in which you can become an expert,
helped by regular use of a variety of mixtures. I suggest the following oils
for room fragrancing and general mood uplift. You can use other oils—be as
creative as you wish. The oils are blended in a carrier.

When oils are blended in the correct ratio, each oil's power is intensified
and all the constituents of the oils work together. The outcome is a blend that
is greater than the sum of its parts. This results in a synergistic effect whereby
the whole mixture works together harmoniously.

You can also use a hot diffuser or an ultrasonic diffuser when creating your
blends, making your own air freshener and room fragrance. With the help of
some well-chosen oils, you will be able to achieve the right mood, reduce stress,
and enjoy the fragrant ambience of your choice.

When vaporized, essential oils
flow through the air and stimulate the
odor receptors located at the base of
the nose. These receptors are directly
connected to the limbic system, the
area responsible for emotions, memory,
and mood. In this way, the essential
oils have the power to affect our moods
and emotions, as well as evoking fond
memories.

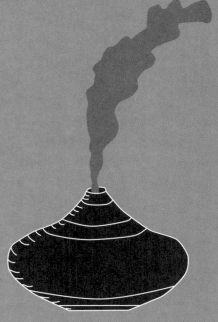

Eastern Magic

Blend aromatics from the East in a carrier of your choice, using warming sandalwood, mystic and captivating patchouli, and exotic ylang-ylang to create a seductive mixture. You can sweeten the mix with a splash of luxurious jasmine instead of one of the three oils mentioned if you wish to further enhance, exhilarate, and seduce the senses.

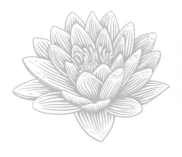

Fruity Refresher

As always, use a carrier of your choice to create this uplifting blend of delicious citrus fruits that smells like a garden orchard. Use a twist of orange and lemon mixed with grapefruit to lift your spirits and refresh you. Alternatively, go further and add a dash of spice to the mixture by enhancing the blend with energizing cinnamon oil. A tantalizing creation!

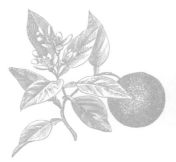

Country Harvest

Make up a rich blend of this medley of flowery oils: geranium, marjoram, and chamomile. It will create a warm pungent aroma, redolent of a warm, sultry summer's day in the countryside. Enjoy this rural creation when you feel the need for therapeutic relaxation.

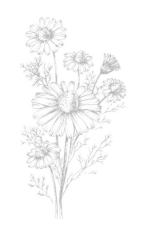

Mindfulness

To get into a meditative mood, create a blend
of bergamot, jasmine, and frankincense. This
will put you in a relaxed mental state, ready for
your session. Frankincense calms and uplifts
simultaneously and it helps concentration.
This oil has been used since biblical times to
promote clarity of mind and spiritual growth.

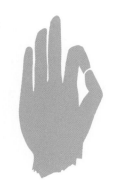

Serenity Moments

When your nerves are frazzled and your
energies are low, regain tranquility and
equilibrium with a blend of clary sage, ylang-
ylang, and vetiver. The sedating and relaxing
aromas of these oils will put you into a deeply
peaceful mood.

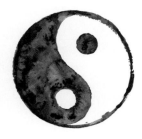

Spice Islands

With a blend of ginger, cinnamon, and
sandalwood, this spicy mix evokes the heady
mental image of a tropical island. It will elevate
the senses with its penetrating warmth. Enjoy
its alluring spicy sweetness whenever you are in
a sensual mood.

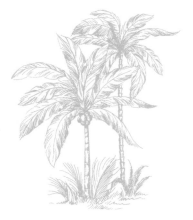

Heavenly Haven

When you want to get away from it all, to enjoy some peace and quiet undisturbed by the sights and sounds of everyday living, visit your own personal sanctuary. Use the comforting fragrance of lavender, orange, and geranium, three oils that work well together, soothing your soul and restoring your energies.

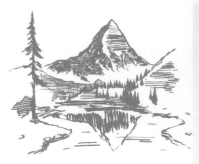

Mind Enhancer

If you need to focus on mental work such as writing, studying, or preparing to take an exam, an inspirational composition of stimulating rosemary, purifying peppermint, and bracing pine will help to lift mental fatigue, improve concentration, and clear your thinking.

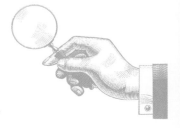

Green Magic

Frankincense and vetiver create a lush and verdant mixture. This resin and grass blend creates an uplifting aroma suitable for any occasion. Add a drop of thyme oil—fresh, green, and herbaceous— to the blend and enjoy the perfumed mist released from your diffuser.

GLOSSARY

Absolute an oil obtained by solvent extraction

Adaptogen promotes homeostasis

Analgesic pain relieving

Antibacterial eliminates bacterial infections

Antidepressant relieves low mood

Antifungal eliminates fungal infections

Anti-inflammatory reduces redness and swelling

Antiseptic infection-fighting substance found in most essential oils

Antispasmodic relieves cramps and spasms

Antiviral stimulates the immune system, helping to eliminate viruses

Astringent tightens tissue

Bactericidal helps to kill bacteria

Carrier oil (base oil) oils made from vegetables, seeds, and nuts that are used to dilute (carry) essential oils

Decongestant relieves congestion

Detoxifying cleanses the system of toxins

Digestive tonic improves digestion

Diuretic increases urinary flow, reducing puffiness caused by fluid retention

Expectorant helps expel phlegm

Febrifuge reduces fever

Hemostatic stems the flow of blood

Homeostasis ability to maintain a state of balance and equilibrium

Hypertensive raises lowered blood pressure

Hypnotic helps induce sleep

Nervine strengthens the nervous system

Sedative calms the nervous system

Stimulant increases activity of the body

Tonic strengthens the body

Toxic poisonous

Vasodilator causes capillaries to expand

ABOUT THE AUTHOR

Marlene Houghton, PhD (Holistic Nutrition)

Marlene Houghton has always been interested in natural health therapies. She has studied herbal healing, holistic nutrition, and related natural therapies, and has learned how they help to keep the body in balance. Marlene has over twenty years' experience working in orthodox medical settings as a medical personal assistant, working with medical doctors in top London teaching hospitals. She is an astrologer, tarot consultant, and tutor. She is also a nutritional therapist and a traditional herbalist.

Marlene is a Consultant Member for the British Astrological and Psychic Society, and, as one of its tutors, she teaches and lectures on various forms of astrology (not all associated with health). She is also a regular contributor of articles on natural health, traditional herbalism, and the way these disciplines link with esoteric traditions for *Mercury* magazine, produced by the British Astrological and Psychic Society. Marlene is a published author. Her first book, *An Astrological Apothecary*, outlines which complementary health methods and natural remedies are compatible with each Sun Sign, and her second, *Herbs for Health*, covers herbalism in a clear and easy manner for a beginner to understand and use.

IMAGE CREDITS

INDEX